PLACEMENT LEARNING IN

Surgical **Nursing**

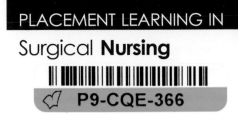

P9-CQE-366

Commissioning Editor: Ninette Premdas/Mairi McCubbin
Development Editor: Sally Davies/Carole McMurray
Project Manager: Andrew Riley
Designer/Design Direction: Charles Gray/Miles Hitchen
Illustration Manager: Jennifer Rose

Placement Learning in

Surgical **Nursing**

A guide for students in practice

Karen Holland BSc(Hons) MSc Cert Ed SRN
Research Fellow, School of Nursing, Midwifery and Social Work, University of Salford, Salford, UK

Michelle Roxburgh Msc, PG Cert LTHE, RGN
Lead for Educational Development Unit, School of Nursing, Midwifery and Health, University of Stirling, Stirling, UK

Series Editor:
Karen Holland BSc(Hons) MSc CertEd SRN
Research Fellow, School of Nursing, Midwifery and Social Work, University of Salford, Salford, UK

Student Adviser:
Philippa Sharp
Student Nurse, Division of Nursing, University of Nottingham, Nottingham, UK

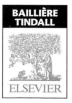

BAILLIÈRE TINDALL

ELSEVIER

Edinburgh   London   New York   Oxford   Philadelphia   St Louis   Sydney   Toronto 2012

BAILLIÈRE
TINDALL
ELSEVIER

ISBN 978-0-7020-4305-5

British Library Cataloguing in Publication Data
A catalogue record for this book is available from the British Library

Library of Congress Cataloging in Publication Data
A catalog record for this book is available from the Library of Congress

Notices
Knowledge and best practice in this field are constantly changing. As new research and experience broaden our understanding, changes in research methods, professional practices, or medical treatment may become necessary.

Practitioners and researchers must always rely on their own experience and knowledge in evaluating and using any information, methods, compounds, or experiments described herein. In using such information or methods they should be mindful of their own safety and the safety of others, including parties for whom they have a professional responsibility.

With respect to any drug or pharmaceutical products identified, readers are advised to check the most current information provided (i) on procedures featured or (ii) by the manufacturer of each product to be administered, to verify the recommended dose or formula, the method and duration of administration, and contraindications. It is the responsibility of practitioners, relying on their own experience and knowledge of their patients, to make diagnoses, to determine dosages and the best treatment for each individual patient, and to take all appropriate safety precautions.

To the fullest extent of the law, neither the Publisher nor the authors, contributors, or editors, assume any liability for any injury and/or damage to persons or property as a matter of products liability, negligence or otherwise, or from any use or operation of any methods, products, instructions, or ideas contained in the material herein.

ELSEVIER your source for books, journals and multimedia in the health sciences

www.elsevierhealth.com

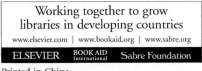

Working together to grow libraries in developing countries

www.elsevier.com | www.bookaid.org | www.sabre.org

ELSEVIER   BOOK AID International   Sabre Foundation

The Publisher's policy is to use **paper manufactured from sustainable forests**

Printed in China

Contents

Section 1
Preparation for practice placement experience 1

Section 2
Placement learning opportunities 59

Contents

Series Preface

Learning to become a nurse is a journey which sees the student engaging in both challenging and life-changing experiences as well as developing their skills and knowledge base in order to be able to practise as a competent and accountable practitioner. To be able to do this requires engagement with others in two different, yet complementary environments, namely the clinical setting and university, with the ultimate aim of learning the necessary knowledge and skills to be able to care for patients, clients and their families in whatever field of practice the student chooses to pursue. The clinical placement becomes the centre of this integrated learning experience.

Tracey Levett-Jones and Sharon Bourgeois (2007) point out, however, that 'there is plenty of evidence, anecdotal and empirical, to suggest that clinical placements can be both tremendous and terrible' but that it is at the same time 'one of the most exciting journeys of your life'. Whilst their book focuses on helping you through this journey in relation to the more 'general' aspects of learning and coping when undertaking your clinical experiences, this series of books sets out to help you gain maximum learning from specific placement-learning opportunities and placements.

The focus of each book is the actual nature of the placements, the client/patient groups you may encounter and the fundamentals of care they might require, together with the evidence-based knowledge and skills that underpin that care. Whilst the general structure of each book might be different, the underpinning principles are the same in each.

To ensure that the learning undertaken in university is linked to that in practice there will be reference to academic regulations, specific learning responsibilities (such as meeting with personal tutors, mentor-student relationships, placement expectations) and the importance of professional accountability.

Each book also outlines how your experiences in practice will help you achieve specific learning outcomes and competencies as specified by the United Kingdom (UK) Nursing and Midwifery Council (NMC). Although the books are primarily aimed at the UK student, the general principles underpinning the care practice described and the underpinning evidence base throughout are valid for all student nurses who are required by their respective international professional organisations to gain experience in a number of clinical environments in order to become competent to practice as a registered qualified nurse.

Nursing is a challenging and rewarding profession. The books in this series offer a foundation of knowledge and learning to support you on your professional journey and their content is based on the editors' and authors' experiences of engaging with students and colleagues in this learning experience. In addition, their content draws on personal experience of working with service users and carers as to what is best practice in caring for people at various stages of life and with various health problems. The ultimate aim is to enable you to use them as 'pocket guides' to learning in a range of clinical placements and specific planned placement learning opportunities, and to share their content with those who manage this learning experience in practice. We hope that you find them a valued resource and companion during your journey to becoming a qualified nurse.

Karen Holland
Series Editor

Student Foreword

Like most students, I have experienced a range of feelings on starting a new placement: the fears and excitement of what experiences you will have, who you are going to meet and work with, what you will learn, and the responsibilities that come with being that bit further along in your training. These are all feelings that are part of our education and training and contribute to the student's growth as a nurse and as an individual. What is expected of you during a placement is another persistent anxiety, in particular, how you can get the best from that specific placement and how you achieve the gold standard of truly incorporating theory into your practice in an effective and useful way.

Most placement experiences vary in length from introductory 2-week placements to full 18-week hub-and-spoke placements. It can take a significant amount of the placement time to settle in, understand the way that particular clinical area works and develop an effective professional relationship with your mentor and other members of staff that enables you to learn and achieve.

This series of books makes the gap between what is taught in the University and practiced in clinical placements much smaller and less frightening. It provides guidance on achieving the Nursing and Midwifery Council (NMC) outcomes and proficiencies, which are essential for becoming a registered nurse, using case studies and real examples to help you. Knowledge of what opportunities to seek in particular clinical areas and how best to achieve them helps considerably, especially when there is so much else to think about. The series also provides a number of opportunities to recap essential knowledge needed for that area (very useful as lectures can seem a long time ago!). From student nurses setting out on that journey to those nearly ending, these books are a valuable resource and support and will help you overcome these sudden panic attacks when you suddenly think 'what do I do now?'. Enjoy them as I have enjoyed being able to have an opportunity to contribute to their development.

Philippa Sharp
3rd Year Student Nurse
University of Nottingham

Student Foreword

Acknowledgements

This book is one of a series written to help student nurses learn from their clinical practice experiences. It will also enable those who both teach and assess this learning to engage with the learning the student is required to achieve by the Nursing and Midwifery Council and the learning outcomes of their graduate programme.

In recognizing this integrated learning and the collaboration involved in making this successful we wish to acknowledge and thank all those students who have helped shape this book, their mentors and numerous other excellent role models and many other health care professionals. We acknowledge that major thanks must go to those patients who the students have met and will meet during their surgical nursing placement. Their journey and that of the students run alongside each other and the case studies in this book reflect this experience.

Personal thanks however must go to the Elsevier team for enabling not only this book to be written and published but also for their invaluable support from idea to publication. We thank Ninette Premdas for her total commitment to the whole series project and for Sally Davies for her support at the beginning of our journey. Mairi McCubbins for her ongoing belief in what we have tried to do and Carole McMurray for her support and cheerfulness. Finally our thanks go to Andrew Riley, whose endless good humour, patience and dedication to his job has enabled us to get to the end!

Section 1. Preparation for practice placement experience

This section focuses on what you need to do and to learn about prior to commencing your surgical nursing placement. There are four chapters, all of which will enable you to gain new knowledge if you have not previously experienced such a placement or update your knowledge if you have.

As well as focusing on general preparation for placement issues which apply to any placement, you will find relevant sections which require active engagement in searching evidence, reading about surgical procedures and, most importantly, anatomy and physiology which is essential for understanding what happens at all stages of a patient's experience of a surgical procedure.

Chapter 1 explains the meaning of surgery and surgical nursing, terminology and key personnel involved in caring for a patient who is undergoing surgery.

Chapter 2 introduces the principles of surgical nursing, explaining the key principles of surgical nursing, knowledge and skills required to care for a patient undergoing surgery and includes some of the evidence base underpinning the principles of surgical nursing.

Chapter 3 explains what a surgical placement is and what you can expect to find in terms of the environment in which perioperative care takes place. It explores some learning opportunities you might experience and also the various kinds of placements where specific types of surgical interventions are carried out.

Chapter 4 focuses on specific learning and/or revision prior to your placement. Short revision points, tests and goal setting for your Nursing and Midwifery Council (NMC) competencies and essential skills are explored.

1

Surgical nursing in context

CHAPTER AIMS

- To introduce the meaning of surgery and surgical nursing
- To introduce various healthcare personnel a student may meet during a surgical placement
- To introduce the terminology a student may come across in relation to surgical nursing
- To identify key learning points to ensure a successful learning experience

Introduction

You are now undertaking a course at a university which will lead to a qualification as a nurse and also an academic award of a diploma or degree. From September 2013, all pre-registration nursing programmes in the UK will be undergraduate degree programmes. The Nursing and Midwifery Council (NMC) which sets out the standards and competencies expected from a qualified nurse also sets out the expected time required for learning in practice. This varies in different countries, but in the UK this has to be 50% of your programme. This 50% can be experienced in many ways, including short visits to learn what happens in such places as the school nurse service or the law courts. These may be part of a theoretical-based module in the university or part of a much longer placement experience. This book mainly focuses upon these longer placement experiences, although different aspects of caring for someone who is undergoing a surgical procedure of any kind are also explored.

Some of you may also experience what is called a 'hub and spoke' placement experience, where you have a base in your main placement but, during the whole of that placement, you may undertake shorter periods of time in other linked areas. Examples of these kinds of placements are found throughout the book.

Depending on the structure and management of your learning experiences in the practice environment and, of course, which field of practice or branch of nursing you are undertaking, you may have a placement which is known as a 'surgical placement'. Most surgical placements are encountered within a hospital, although you may see surgical procedures and care in other contexts such as a health centre.

What is surgery ?

Before we determine what a surgical placement is, it is important to determine what we mean by surgical and surgery. The term 'surgical' implies some kind of surgery which involves an *operative* or *invasive intervention* – an operation normally involves 'cutting into' various parts of the body. An example is removal of the gall bladder through a laparoscope, which is a long, thin telescope with a light and camera lens at the tip which is passed through a number of small cuts in the abdomen but doesn't involve large wounds. This allows the surgeon (the doctor who performs the surgery) to view the internal organs on a monitor. Surgery may be *exploratory* and *diagnostic*, or it may be life-saving following a serious *life-threatening trauma*. Although the principles of surgery remain the same, the way in which surgery is carried out has changed significantly. A brief overview of the development of surgery over time will enable you to understand why some patients may be frightened of undergoing any kind of invasive procedure and also why some procedures, such as removing sutures from some surgical wounds, are no longer carried out following surgery due to advances both in surgical techniques and technology.

Brief history of surgery

Although there is evidence of various types of what we would call surgical procedures taking place in the Middle Ages and before, for the purpose of this overview we focus on the nineteenth century onwards (1800 to the present day) and the images that many of us will have seen in relation to early surgical work, such as amputation without anaesthetic, management of pain or dying due to wound infection.

An excellent overview of the history of surgery over time can be found on the Channel 4 website: http://www.channel4. com/explore/surgerylive/history.html. As well as specific information about surgery generally, this site also has short videos of patients talking about their experiences of surgery and why it was necessary, for example a patient who underwent surgery for a pituitary tumour (http://www. channel4.com/explore/surgerylive/ surgical4.html). This website also offers an insight into some of the roles of individuals during the intraoperative period, and in these short videos there are visual images of what the environment in an operating room or anaesthetic room is like.

Surgery today is, of course, very different due to advances both in surgical techniques and what we know about the human body. The most common cause of death after surgery used to be infection, but following the initial findings of Louis Pasteur (that the death of body tissue was due to bacteria in the air) and Ignaz Semmelweis (who discovered that 'transmission of infectious diseases could be reduced by handwashing' (Kozier et al 2008:644)), Joseph Lister, a British surgeon, introduced the use of carbolic acid and other antiseptic techniques 'to kill bacteria in his operating theatres' (Kozier et al 2008). Effective hand washing, as part of the much wider infection control agenda, is one of the key skills that you will need as a student and qualified nurse, not only in a surgical placement but every placement.

Alongside these discoveries and practices was the introduction of anaesthetic during surgery, early ones being ether and chloroform, which subsequently led to the more sophisticated techniques and preparations in use today (see Ch. 7).

Types of surgery

There are two main types of surgery: emergency and elective. Kozier et al (2008:644) define these as follows:

> *Emergency surgery is performed immediately to preserve function or the*

life of the patient. Surgeries to control internal haemorrhage or repair a fracture are examples of emergency surgeries. Elective surgery is performed when surgical intervention is the preferred treatment for a condition that is not imminently life threatening (but may ultimately threaten life or well-being) or to improve the patient's life. Examples of elective surgeries include cholecystectomy for chronic gall bladder disease, hip replacement surgery or plastic surgery procedures such as breast reduction surgery.

Activity

Access the website of the Royal College of Surgeons of England, for general information on different types of surgery:
http://www.rcseng.ac.uk/patient_information/faqs/different_surgery.html (accessed December 2011).

You will find a number of resources that you might find useful prior to starting your clinical placement. Access the patient information section and consider how the information will help you to explain to a patient their journey through an elective surgery.
The following is a link to a guide to help teams make the most of a patient's journey through elective surgery (Patient Liaison Group/RCSE 2007):
http://www.rcseng.ac.uk/publications/docs/patient_journey.html (accessed December 2011).

In addition to the two different types of surgery, there are two further subdivisions, namely major and minor. Major surgery involves a bigger risk to the patient, not only in terms of the organs of the body that may be involved but the intricacy of the surgery and possible postoperative complications that may occur (see Ch. 12). An example of this is a heart and lung transplant.

Minor surgery can also be intricate, but there is less risk and fewer complications. This kind of surgery is usually undertaken as 'day care surgery' (see Ch. 11). An example of this is removal of a skin lesion.

Reflection point

You might meet nurse practitioners who have undertaken specialised training to undertake minor surgical procedures (see Martin 2002) and choose to spend a day observing their work as part of your main placement experience.

Surgical nursing placement

During your course, you may be allocated to a placement in an environment where surgery takes place. In the main, this will be in a hospital; however, more and more healthcare practices are now undertaking minor surgical procedures and you may be able to gain some experience of the basic principles of surgical intervention in a community placement.

For the purpose of this book, we consider a surgical placement as an area within a hospital where operative or invasive interventions take place. A nursing term often used in relation to surgery is 'perioperative care', which involves caring for the patient before admission to hospital, during the admission process, preoperative care (i.e. prior to going to the operating theatre), care during the operation and postoperative care (both immediately and until discharge home). The learning of principles underpinning these stages is transferrable to other placements where you may encounter a surgical procedure but where the focus of care for the patients is not surgery.

Surgical nursing, therefore, involves caring for patients throughout their perioperative journey. To care for patients during this time requires both general and specific knowledge and skills, depending on the nature of the surgical intervention and the individual needs of the patient. A knowledge of the following is required:

- The principles of surgical nursing.
- Normal and abnormal physiological processes and illnesses.
- Anatomy.
- Pharmacology.
- Management of pain.
- Diagnostic tests.
- Surgical procedures.
- Risks and complications of surgery for different age groups.
- Most importantly, effective assessment, goal setting and planning, implementing and evaluating care delivered.

See Chapter 2 for further information regarding preparation prior to undertaking a surgical placement. Also, access specific placement learning information relevant to your local NHS organisations on your university website.

Healthcare personnel on a surgical placement

As well as nurses with various titles, you will come across a number of other healthcare personnel while on a surgical placement. Table 1.1 lists those you might encounter in the preoperative period (some of whom you may also meet in a pre-admission clinic), with a brief summary of their roles. Tables 1.2 and 1.3 list those you might encounter during the intraoperative and postoperative periods, respectively, some of whom you will see at every stage of a patient's journey.

Activity

What do the terms preoperative and postoperative mean? How would you explain these to a relative who asked you what they meant, after telling you they were going into hospital for an operation?

You will find some of the answers in this chapter.

Explaining terminology that is unfamiliar to patients is a key aspect of your role and is an important communication skill. This activity could form the basis of a goal in relation to achieving competence in communicating effectively with patients and their relatives (NMC Standard 2010: Domain–Communication and Interpersonal Skills: NMC Standard 2004: Domain–Care Delivery).

Activity

Make a list of all the members of the surgical team and find out as much about their roles as possible prior to starting your placement.

Work out which of the roles you would like to find out more about during the placement. Discuss with your mentor on arrival the possibility of spending time with at least two of these during your placement to understand more about how they contribute to the care of the patients you will be nursing.

For example, you may be asked as part of an assignment to consider various roles during your placement and discuss how they have made a contribution to a patient in your care (interprofessional working). Make notes from your observations of their role and invite them to explain how this contributes to the care given (this must be under the supervision and agreement of your mentor).

Terminology related to care for patients undergoing a surgical procedure

Students reading this introduction will already be considering the meaning of some of the terminology used, which will underpin much of what we discuss in Sections 2 and 3. It is essential that, prior to beginning your placement, you become familiar with some of these terms, as this will help you to understand what nurses and other professionals are talking about when discussing patient care as well as allowing you to explain them to patients and their families.

Table 1.1 Roles of healthcare personnel in the preoperative period

Named role	Role description and responsibilities
Qualified registered nurse	A person who has been approved by the NMC as being 'fit for practice' at the end of a course of study and who has met all the NMC Standards and Competencies for Registration as a Nurse
Ward sister/manager/charge nurse	A senior nurse who is responsible for the immediate management and leadership of a group of staff, together with overall management of the patients in their care This will include clinical leadership in a specific field of practice
Specialist nurses such as pain management nurse, infection control nurse	A specialist nurse is someone who has a senior clinical role in an organisation and has developed their knowledge and skills to an advanced level in a particular area of clinical care and offers additional expertise in the care of a patient
Radiographer	A person who has undertaken a course of study to enable them to register as a radiographer, who takes images of various internal parts of the body as well as undertaking some investigative tests These include X-ray images, computed tomography (CT) scans and magnetic resonance imaging (MRI)
Anaesthetist	A qualified doctor who has specialised in the giving of anaesthetics and managing the care of the patient while anaesthetised There are also nurse anaesthetists who have undergone advanced training to manage the care of patients in certain situations and they work under the guidance of the anaesthetist
Physiotherapist	A person who has undertaken a course of study to register as a physiotherapist, who treats patients with musculoskeletal problems/physical problems in the main, with activity and other therapies

Continued

Table 1.1 Roles of healthcare personnel in the preoperative period—cont'd

Named role	Role description and responsibilities
Phlebotomist	A person who is a qualified technician trained to take blood from a patient in order that it can be tested as part of a diagnosis
Social worker	A person who has undertaken a course of study to register as a social worker, who specialises in social, emotional and financial support to individuals and/or families and liaises with other professionals in ensuring effective discharge home from hospital

Table 1.2 Roles in the intraoperative period (adapted from Alexander et al 2006:915)

Named role	Role description and responsibilities
Anaesthetic nurse	Receives the patient in the reception area of the anaesthetic room and checks details Key role is to help relieve patient anxiety prior to surgery
Anaesthetist	Visits patients preoperatively to ensure they understand what is going to happen, if they are fit for an anaesthetic and to prescribe premedication They manage the giving of the anaesthesia and monitor the patient's condition during surgery as well as prescribing postoperative analgesia
Circulating nurse	This is the nurse who manages a range of roles in the theatre, from managing equipment, supporting the scrub nurse, helping to position the patient, cleaning and sterilising any equipment and, most importantly, ensuring safety with regards to instruments and swabs
Scrub nurse	Has a key role in assisting the surgeon; protects the patient's dignity and should be the patient's advocate during the surgery Ensures safety with regards to instruments and swabs and prevents diathermy and pressure injuries
Recovery nurse	Has a key role in the recovery room, ensuring safety and care of the patient in the immediate postoperative period Ensures patency of airway, undertakes essential observations, assesses pain and nausea and gives medication for both according to the prescription Key role in ensuring total patient care, including reassurance, reducing anxiety and maintaining appropriate documentation and communication with ward staff and surgical team involved in the surgery

Table 1.2 Roles in the intraoperative period (adapted from Alexander et al 2006:915)—cont'd

Named role	Role description and responsibilities
Consultant surgeon	*A consultant surgeon is a registered medical practitioner who has undergone approved training and acquired appropriate experience in a surgical specialty such as to allow entry on to the UK Specialist Register and who has been appointed by a recognised procedure such as an Advisory Appointment Committee to provide a surgical service as part of a clinical team. The consultant surgeon, in providing this service, is expected to manage the main condition of the patient, but recognise the need to call in others from the same or different specialties at his or her discretion; to delegate clinical and administrative responsibility at his or her discretion; and to act as the advocate of the patient in relation to their treatment and wellbeing. (RCS 2009;1)*
Registrar (surgical)	A registrar is normally a surgeon who has undertaken a period of about 6 years in a surgical field under the supervision of a consultant They choose an area to specialise in or become a general surgeon, able to carry out a range of surgery To achieve consultant status requires further exams and membership as a Fellow of the Royal College of Surgeons (FRCS)

Table 1.3 Roles in post operative period, including post-discharge home

Named role	Role description and responsibilities
Registered (ward) nurse	A nurse who has undertaken a programme of learning in practice and Higher Education and successfully attained registration as a nurse with the Nursing and Midwifery Council. The nurse can be newly qualified or have extensive experience and expertise in caring for patients who have surgical intervention. This nurse is often either the main nurse for the patient, the nurse in charge of the ward or a specialist nurse focusing on helping the patient with managing pain for example or works in a specialist field such as breast cancer care.
District nurse	*District nurses play a crucial role in the primary health care team. They visit people in their own homes or in residential care homes, providing care for patients and supporting family members.*

Continued

Table 1.3 Roles in post-operative period, including post-discharge home—cont'd

Named role	Role description and responsibilities
	As well as providing direct patient care, district nurses also have a teaching role, working with patients to enable them to care for themselves or with family members teaching them how to give care to their relatives. District nurses play a vital role in keeping hospital admissions and readmissions to a minimum and ensuring that patients can return to their own homes as soon as possible (NHS Careers, http://www.nhscareers.nhs.uk/details/Default.aspx?Id= 916%20)
Health visitor	*A health visitor is a qualified and registered nurse or midwife who has undertaken further (post registration) training in order to be able to work as a member of the primary healthcare team. The role of the health visitor is about the promotion of health and the prevention of illness in all age groups (NHS Careers, http://www.nhscareers.nhs. uk/details/Default.aspx?Id=807)*
Healthcare assistant	*Healthcare assistants can work within hospital or community settings under the guidance of a qualified healthcare professional. The role can be very varied depending upon the area in which the person is employed. Working alongside nurses, for example, they may sometimes be known as nursing auxiliaries or auxiliary nurses. Healthcare assistants also work alongside qualified midwives in maternity services.* *The types of duties include the following:* • *washing and dressing* • *feeding* • *helping people to mobilise* • *toileting* • *bed making* • *generally assisting with patients overall comfort* • *monitoring patients conditions by taking temperatures, pulse, respiration's and weight* *(NHS Careers, http://www.nhscareers.nhs.uk/details/Default.aspx? Id=807)*

Let us look initially at some of the key broad terms used in this book.

Pre-admission Patients who are to attend hospital for surgery, or to undergo a minor surgical procedure in a community health centre, will require information on what is going to happen to them beforehand, in order to reduce anxiety (Walker 2002, Kielty 2008).

Preoperative Preoperative literally means before operation (surgery). Normally this term is used after admission to hospital for a surgical procedure, whether elective or emergency surgery. There are key steps that must be taken before surgery of any kind (see Ch. 5).

Perioperative This term means before (pre-), during (intra-) and immediately after (post-) surgery and usually refers to interventions during those periods (Pudner 2010).

Postoperative Postoperative care takes place in the immediate period after surgery and the period until the patient is discharged home from hospital. It could be argued that the time after a patient is home from hospital until the surgeon decides they no longer need to be seen should also be termed postoperative.

Anaesthetic room For many patients undergoing surgery, an anaesthetic (given by injection or through inhaling as a gas) is required to prevent any painful physical sensations while the invasive procedure is carried out. Anaesthesia can be achieved either locally or generally, as it is not always necessary for a patient to be unconscious during an operation. The anaesthetic room is usually situated next to the operating theatre (Stewart & Huntington 2007).

Theatre The theatre is sometimes known as the 'operating room' and is a very specific organised space which is immediately identified as being the place where surgery takes place. It is also an area that must be free from the possibility of causing infection (sterile environment).

Recovery room Patients having undergone a general anaesthetic require a varied period of time in which to recover safely prior to returning to the ward area. This takes place in the recovery room, where nurses and other healthcare personnel undertake close observation of the patient for any immediate effects of the surgery and anaesthetic.

✔ Tip

Remember to explain abbreviations and avoid their overuse. Also avoid using nursing 'jargon' in your nursing assignments.

↻ Activity

Prior to your placement, check your university practice placement information site (which might look like that in Box 1.1) where you may find examples of types of surgery such as those in Table 1.4. Your university may only be accessible via the Intranet and you will require your own password

If there are new terms for your particular placement, make a list of these and consult a surgical textbook or nursing dictionary to find out their meaning and make a note in your pre-placement notes to discuss with your mentor (see Ch. 3 for more information about this).

Discharge from hospital It is important to consider what will happen or needs to happen for patients once their surgery (minor or major) is over, and the decision about this (i.e. going home from hospital) should be made both before and at admission (NHS Institute for Innovation and Improvement 2008).

Table 1.4 lists some more commonly used terms you will encounter on a surgical placement. Other terms are defined and discussed at other points throughout the book, in particular the use of abbreviations commonly used by nurses and the inherent dangers associated with this.

Word meanings
- -ectomy at the end of a word implies 'surgical removal of'.
- -plasty means 'refashioning' or 'plastic repair of'.
- -ostomy means surgically creating an opening connecting the internal organ(s) with the external surface of the body.
- -oscopy means looking inside/ looking into.

Table 1.4 Surgical terminology and meanings (examples only)

Surgical terminology	Meaning
Cholecystectomy	Removal of the gall bladder
Thyroidectomy	Removal of the thyroid gland
Angioplasty	An operation to repair a damaged blood vessel or unblock a coronary artery
Tracheostomy	An opening in the trachea which can be surgically created to ensure a safe airway through inserting a tube
Transurethral resection of bladder	A procedure used to diagnose bladder cancer and remove unusual growths or tumours on the bladder wall The bladder is approached via the actual urethra See: http://hcd2.bupa.co.uk/fact_sheets/htmt/turbt.html
Nephrectomy	Removal of a kidney
Cystoscopy	Examination of the bladder using an instrument called a cystoscope See: http://www.patient.co.uk/health/Cystoscopy.htm
Hysterectomy	Removal of the uterus
Bilateral salpingo-oophorectomy	Removal of both ovaries and fallopian tubes
Amputation	Removal of part of the body, either surgically or by trauma Usually a limb or part of a limb
Arthroplasty	Reconstruction (refashioning) of a new movable joint, e.g. total hip replacement
Laminectomy	Removal of part of a vertebral bone called the lamina in the lower spine
Craniotomy	A cut into the cranium where a temporary bone flap is made into the skull, either to relieve pressure or to access parts of the brain
Tonsillectomy	Removal of the tonsils
Laryngectomy	Removal of the larynx
Oesophagectomy	Removal of the oesophagus
Pancreatectomy	Removal of the pancreas
Gastrectomy	Removal of the stomach
Hemicolectomy	Removal of part of the large bowel

Table 1.4 Surgical terminology and meanings (examples only) — cont'd

Surgical terminology	Meaning
Ileostomy	Making a surgical opening in the abdomen and raising a part of the small bowel, the ileum, onto the surface Usually for serious digestive problems such as cancer of the bowel See: http://www.nhsinform.co.uk/health-library/articles/i/ileostomy/introduction.aspx
Abdominoperineal excision of rectum (colostomy)	An operation where the anus, rectum and sigmoid colon are removed (usually for cancer)
Appendicectomy	Removal of the appendix
Haemorrhoidectomy	Removal of haemorrhoids
Cystectomy	Removal of the bladder
Prostatectomy	Removal of the prostate gland
Vasectomy	The vas deferens (tubes through which sperm travel to the semen) are tied off as contraception See: http://hcd2.bupa.co.uk/fact_sheets/html/vasectomy.html#anim
Laparoscopy	A procedure to look into the abdomen by making small cuts and inserting a laparoscope See: http://www.patient.co.uk/health/Laparoscopy-and-Laparoscopic-surgery.htm
Colporrhaphy	A surgical repair of a prolapse deficit in the vaginal wall See: http://hcd2.bupa.co.uk/fact_sheets/html/qanda/vaginal_repair_surgery_qanda.html
Mastectomy	Removal of the breast See: http://hcd2.bupa.co.uk/fact_sheets/html/vaginal_repair_surgery_qanda.html

Box 1.1 Example of a clinical placement website for students

Clinical placement

Intensive Care Unit (ICU), Ravenscourt Hospitals NHS Trust (pseudonym), London Road, Manchester

Description

A 28-bed female orthopaedic surgical ward

Continued

Box 1.1 Example of a clinical placement website for students—cont'd

Your contact(s)

Michelle Roxburgh: e-mail: XXX

Further information can be obtained via telephone/address: XXX

Your university contact

Karen Holland: e-mail: XXX

What is organised for students on commencement of placement?

- A session on the role of the practice education team including mentors and practice education facilitators.
- All students will be given a welcome letter with the name of their main mentor and all members of the main multidisciplinary team.
- Whenever possible, and in accordance with NMC requirements, the student and mentor will work together throughout the placement and off duty will be coordinated to reflect this.
- An introduction booklet (containing detailed information about the ward and orthopaedic surgical nursing, including a brief outline of nursing procedures and observations that students can engage in under direct and indirect supervision) will also be given on arrival and discussed in the first interview with the named mentor.

What are the arrangements for mentors and students?

Students will be allocated a mentor, usually on arrival, who will undertake the main assessor role. It is envisioned that you will mostly work with your mentor, but supporting learning in practice is a team effort and, as such, the main mentor will discuss student progress with a range of other members of the healthcare team.

What shift patterns are students allocated for learning?

- Early: 07.30–15.30 with half hour break
- Late: 13.00–21.00 with half hour (unpaid) break as per trust policy
- Night: 20.30–07.30
- 07.30–21.00 with 1 hour break (long day shift)

Long day shifts are optional for students. Students are required to undertake their learning to experience the whole 24-hour care of patients and night duty is arranged in relation to your goals for the placement and requirements of your programme.

If you are going to be late or are sick, you must contact the ward at the first opportunity.

What patient care situations are available in this placement?

Students are involved in pre- and postoperative care for patients undergoing joint replacements, arthrodesis, arthroscopes and other elective orthopaedic surgery.

Box 1.1 Example of a clinical placement website for students—cont'd

What nursing model is used for planning care?

The Roper, Logan and Tierney model, adapted for the specific needs of patients undergoing elective orthopaedic surgery.

What core clinical skills can be learnt?

Generally, students can gain experience in the following:

■ A systematic approach to patient assessment, planning, implementing and evaluating care (holistic care).
■ A good foundation in physiological knowledge and how to measure a patient's progress through clinical measurements.
■ Aseptic technique for wounds.
■ Dressing application.
■ Insertion/removal of urinary catheters.
■ Care of venflon sites and intravenous infusions.
■ Removal of sutures/clips.
■ Removal of wound drains.
■ Observations pre- and postoperatively.
■ Use of patient-controlled analgesia (PCA).
■ Epidurals.
■ Discharge planning.

What additional clinical skills can be learnt?

Care of patients undergoing joint replacement surgery, including the patient journey through perioperative care such as in the anaesthetic room, recovery and the actual theatre, and key skills that can be learnt in each area. Airway management is a major skill.

What resources are available to help learning?

■ Organised, planned teaching sessions: teaching packs are available with a focus on key types of management of the care of patients undergoing orthopaedic surgery.
■ A wide range of nursing journals and access to the NHS trust library and computer databases.
■ A wealth of experienced staff who are keen to make the student's experience a positive one: discussion with mentor about learning goals.
■ Students are actively encouraged to attend the NHS trust acute care study sessions for all staff after discussion with their mentor.

What research and practice development activities are being undertaken?

Two members of the ward team are investigating postoperative wound care and infection control procedures.

✔ **Tip**

A useful tip is to keep a notebook for use at home and at university. Make notes about the care of patients undergoing various surgical interventions, why they are having the surgery, what signs and symptoms they had been experiencing prior to surgery, what the nursing management was and any general aspects of care. Alternatively, you might keep notes in a ring-binder file and add articles you have found related to various aspects of care or underpinning physiology, etc. Add notes about medications patients have received – this is essential because, as a qualified nurse, you will be expected to know most of the 'basic' drugs, their side effects and correct dosages. This is a useful tip for all placements as it helps to build up a collection of notes which you can use to share with others or as a record of learning for your portfolios.

◐ **Activity**

During your surgical placement, make a list in your notes of all the different types of surgical interventions you come across. A list of some of these may already be available on the university placement website.

Find out what each one involves and make notes on the signs and symptoms patients requiring this surgery may be experiencing and also the care they require following the procedure. Use an up-to-date textbook to help you with this. This will begin to focus your learning in preparation for the placement and help you to set goals with your mentor with regards to total patient care experiences.

Although most students undergoing surgical placements may be from either an adult or child health field of practice (branch), some students from mental health and learning disability fields of practice may also experience this placement. Also, patients in these latter fields of practice may have to be admitted to hospital for a surgical procedure and it would be an excellent learning experience for the student caring for them to consider an opportunity for following the total patient pathway. Discuss it with your mentor if this occurs while you are undertaking a placement in either a mental health or learning disabilities field of practice.

References

Alexander, M., Fawcett, J.N., Runciman, P.J., 2006. Nursing practice: hospital and home: the adult. Churchill Livingstone, Edinburgh.

Kielty, L.A., 2008. An investigation into the information received by patients undergoing a gastroscopy in a large teaching hospital in Ireland. Gastroenterology Nursing 31 (3), 212–222.

Kozier, B., Erb, G., Berman, A., et al., 2008. Fundamentals of nursing – concepts, process and practice. Pearson Education, Harlow.

Martin, S., 2002. Developing the nurse practitioner's role in minor surgery. Nursing Times 98 (33), 39–40.

NHS Institute for Innovation and Improvement, 2008. Discharge planning. NHS, London. Online. Available at: http://www.institute.nhs.uk/quality_ and_service_improvement_tools/ quality_and_service_improvement_ tools/discharge_planning.html (accessed September 2011).

Patient Liaison Group, 2007. Improving your patient elective journey. Royal College of Surgeons, London.

Pudner, R. (Ed.), 2010. Nursing the surgical patient, third ed. Baillière Tindall, Edinburgh.

Stewart, L., Huntington, S., 2007. The peri-operative phase. In: McArthur-Rouse, F., Prosser, S. (Eds.), Assessing and managing the acutely ill adult surgical patient. Blackwell, Oxford: 17–38.

Walker, J.A., 2002. Emotional and psychological preoperative preparation in adults. British Journal of Nursing 11 (8), 567–575.

Further reading

Brooker, C., Waugh, A., 2007. Foundations of nursing practice. Mosby, Edinburgh.

McArthur-Rouse, F., Prosser, S., 2007. Assessing and managing the acutely ill adult surgical patient. Blackwell, Oxford.

Waugh, A., Grant, A., 2010. Ross and Wilson anatomy and physiology in health and illness, 11th ed. Churchill Livingstone, Edinburgh.

Websites

For an insight into the role of the anaesthetist: http://www.nhs.uk/conditions/anaesthetic-general/Pages/Definition.aspx (accessed December 2011).

For an explanation of different roles in the NHS: http://www.nhscareers.nhs.uk/career.shtml (accessed December 2011).

For those of you undertaking a surgical experience in a children's ward or visiting as part of a 'hub and spoke' placement learning opportunity, there are two publications linked to children's experience of surgery available on the Royal College of Surgeons website: http://www.rcseng.ac.uk/publications/docs/going-into-hospital-for-an-operation and http://www.rcseng.ac.uk/publications/docs/children_hospital.html (accessed December 2011).

2

Introduction to the principles of surgical nursing

CHAPTER AIMS

- To consider the key principles of surgical nursing
- To determine what knowledge and skills the student will need to understand and be able to undertake in order to care for a patient requiring surgery
- To consider the evidence base underpinning aspects of surgical nursing

The key principles of surgical nursing

We saw in Chapter 1 that there are key words associated with surgery, where it takes place and the roles of various healthcare professionals in the care of patients and their families. Given that you will be learning and working alongside qualified nurses who will be your mentors, it is essential that you familiarise yourself with key aspects of care that a nurse may be involved with.

In this chapter, we provide an overview of the main responsibilities of the nurse in relation to key areas of practice in a surgical placement, and help you to identify what knowledge and skills you will need to ensure best evidence-based practice and patient care. It is important, as with any placement, that you undertake some preliminary reading with regards to patient care, including normal physiology, and, if possible, update some of the key clinical skills required in a surgical placement. The chapter helps you understand how to achieve the NMC Competencies and Essential Skills relevant to your learning experience in a surgical placement, as well as identifying recommended reading prior to the placement. This also helps you to develop your evidence-based practice, an essential part of becoming a competent practitioner on completion of your programme of study (see Ch. 4).

The key areas are the following:

- Assessment, planning, implementing and evaluating care using a nursing model or framework.
- Managing fluid and electrolyte balance.
- Managing nutrition.
- Managing pain.
- Managing infection control.
- Managing wounds and wound care.
- Managing stress and anxiety.
- Managing possible altered body image.

It is important to remember that every patient you meet is an individual and so all those you care for during the perioperative period will be unique in their previous experience of hospital, their present illness and their full medical history. It is possible, however, to identify key aspects of care that will be the same for all patients admitted to hospital for surgery.

Assessment, planning, implementing and evaluating care using a nursing model or framework

Admission to hospital, whether it is for a day or longer, is a potentially stressful and anxious experience for patients as well as for their families (Walker 2002). This is one of the main reasons why ensuring patients receive preoperative information about their surgery and their stay in hospital is so important. The development of pre-admission assessment prior to a stay in hospital has become increasingly utilised by the surgical team, which includes nurses as well as surgeons and anaesthetists working together (Fisher & McMillan 2004). This topic is considered in more detail in Chapter 5.

In this chapter, we cover the general principles of assessment of patients, along with planning, implementing and evaluating care; in other words the nursing process as a framework for helping you to learn to care for patients when you begin your placement experience. For some of you, this will be revisiting prior knowledge and experience. Not every surgical ward has a care plan document which clearly states that a nursing model is being used (e.g. Roper, Logan and Tierney's activities of living model [Roper et al 2000]). However, as a student, using the principles of a model helps you to develop a set of skills and knowledge about how to assess, plan, implement and evaluate care as well as focusing on helping you identify gaps in your knowledge and practice. In addition to a nursing model as a framework for applying the nursing process, you also need to be aware of the care delivery model

used to deliver care to patients in the surgical placement: for example, is it a team nursing approach or primary nursing?

Activity

Find out which nursing model is used in your placement as a framework for care, and if no specific one appears to be used, consider how you could use one to help you learn to assess a patient on admission to hospital and identify needs prior to surgery. (An example of a nursing care plan document can be found in Appendix 3 in Holland et al (2008), as well as a list of questions you may need to ask patients to help ensure best practice and patient safety.) All students need to be able to use a method such as the nursing process to enable them to identify and meet the needs of patients. For those pursuing the adult nursing field of practice (previously known as a branch), the NMC Standards and Competencies in Box 2.1 are particularly relevant.

Paper to read prior to placement:

Shirey M R (2008) Nursing practice models for acute and critical care: an overview of care delivery models. Critical Care Nursing Clinics of North America 20(4):365–373.

Although this paper is written in the context of a US healthcare system, it is applicable to the UK NHS and compares a range of care delivery options that you will come across in your placements.

Managing fluid and electrolyte balance

Major surgery of any kind will involve a certain amount of blood or fluid loss. To be able to understand what is happening to a

---

Box 2.1 Examples of NMC Standards and Competencies (NMC 2010)

Domain: Nursing Practice and Decision Making

Field Standard for Competence (Adult Nursing)

Adult nurses must also be able to carry out accurate health, clinical and nursing assessments across all ages and show the right diagnostic and decision-making skills. They must have the confidence to provide effective adult nursing care in the home, the community and in hospital settings to individuals and communities. They must be able to respond to a range of healthcare needs and levels of dependency including: immediate care, critical care, acute care, intermediate care, long-term conditions, palliative care and end of life care.

Competencies

Generic

1. *All nurses must work loosely with individuals, groups and carers, using a range of skills to carry out comprehensive, systematic and holistic assessments. These must take into account current and previous physical, social, cultural, psychological, spiritual, genetic and environmental factors that may be relevant to the individual and their families.*

  1.1. *Adult nurses must safely use a range of diagnostic and clinical skills, complemented by existing and developing technology, to assess the nursing care of individuals undergoing therapeutic or clinical interventions.*

Field Specific

2.2. *Adult nurses must develop and use care pathways and care plans, recognising when standard care pathways are inappropriate and when care should be tailored to individual needs and circumstances. They must understand the physical and psychological impact of long-term conditions, lifestyle, health needs or periods of acute illness. They must then adjust nursing interventions to take account of when people have more than one health need or condition and a person's ability to care for themselves.*

5.1. *Adult nurses must recognise the early signs of acute illness in young people, adults and older people and accurately assess and start appropriate and timely management of those at risk of clinical deterioration, who are acutely ill or who need emergency care.*

---

patient (with an underpinning knowledge of why this will have an impact on their body) and therefore be able to care for them, it is essential that you understand the management of fluid and electrolytes.

It is part of your role as a student, under the supervision of your mentor, to ensure that a fluid balance chart is maintained and be able to interpret this accurately in order to ensure a patient's internal environment is safe.

It is beyond the scope of this book to cover everything you will need to know and we encourage you to read a physiology textbook which explains the way in which the body normally manages fluid and electrolyte balance.

Water is essential to human life, and can be found both within and outwith cells. It makes up around 70% of our total body weight and varies from morning to night by around 2% depending on what we have had to eat or drink (Kindlen 2003). To maintain a balance, it is excreted in urine, faeces, skin and sweat and also exhaled from the lungs.

It is essential to maintain the right 'ingredients' in the right amount to manage this balance between enough, too little or too much water. This is why electrolytes are so important in their correct balance. The electrolytes are sodium, potassium and chloride and we consider these in more detail below.

In order to maintain the body's homeostasis (balancing the state of the body's internal environment), different systems have to work together, but for a patient who is ill or has had surgery, this balance may no longer be maintained and signs and symptoms of this will appear. Early detection of these is part of your role as a nurse, and as a student you will need to learn skills and knowledge of how to detect potential problems with fluid balance and thus the balance of electrolytes (see Ch. 20 in Gobbi et al 2006 for a detailed evidence-based approach).

Such skills and knowledge are transferable to other placements, and you may already have experience of detecting possible problems from other placements, which will give you confidence in applying these skills to your surgical placement.

So, how can you be a detective? First, consider Table 2.1 which highlights the different signs and symptoms associated with fluid and electrolyte problems.

✔ Tip

Ensuring you are familiar with how fluid and electrolyte balance works will support your achievement of many NMC Essential Skills and Competencies. For example, as an Essential Skill at Progression Point 2 (probably at the end of year 2) on the NMC regulations (NMC 2010:131), it is expected that:

'People can trust a newly registered graduate nurse to assess and monitor their fluid status and, in partnership with them, formulate an effective care plan:

1. *Applies knowledge of fluid requirements needed for health and during illness and recovery, so that appropriate fluids can be provided.*
2. *Accurately monitors and records fluid intake and output.*
3. *Recognises and reports reasons for poor fluid intake and output.*
4. *Reports to other members of the team when intake and output fall below requirements.'*

We will return to how you can manage learning opportunities to achieve these later in the book.

Paper to read prior to placement:

Castledine G (2003) Nurse who did not keep accurate fluid balance records and was rude. British Journal of Nursing 12(12):717 (accessed December 2011).

Managing nutrition

There is clear evidence that patients can become malnourished in hospital (Edwards 1998, Brogden 2004). The majority of patients undergoing elective

Table 2.1 Signs and symptoms associated with fluid and electrolyte problems

Fluid and electrolyte intake	What could happen and your observations of the effect of this on a fluid balance chart as well as personal observation of the patient
A patient has not drunk anything for 12 hours and has been vomiting (they are not being given any intravenous fluid at this time).	If the patient has not been drinking any fluids but is also losing fluid, this means that fluid loss is exceeding intake. This will cause the patient to become dehydrated. You will be able to see this on a fluid balance chart and it is important to measure the amount of vomit if possible (i.e. if the patient has vomited into a vomit bowl and it is mainly liquid, this can be measured). The body will also respond by trying to conserve fluid, and therefore there will be a reduction in urine output, which you will also note on the chart. If this persists without treatment, additional signs will become apparent but these will be visible through personal observation of the patient rather than on the fluid balance chart. It is important to monitor both.
An elderly lady has returned from the operating theatre and is not having any oral fluids. Due to lack of close observation of her intravenous fluid intake, she has absorbed 1 litre over 15 minutes instead of the 6 hours prescribed.	Obviously, it is essential that any patient returning from theatre should be closely observed for signs of physiological and other changes. This is part of the NMC Code (NMC 2009) However, occasionally, and for valid reasons such as positioning of the arm or restlessness of the patient, IV fluids may 'run through' the tubing at a faster rate than it should If this does happen, it could have serious consequences due to circulatory overload, especially if the patient is elderly or there is another underlying health problem where a sudden overload of fluid is not advisable. It is important to notify the doctor in charge of the patient's care initially, who will advise certain protocols and also close observation of the patient. Key signs of fluid overload include tachycardia, raised blood pressure, wheezing or other signs of respiratory distress. There may also be restlessness.
A man has returned from theatre having lost a great amount of blood and the surgeon has ordered 4 units of blood to be given over 24 hours. He has already received 2 units of blood in theatre.	During blood transfusion, key observations to make are pulse rate, blood pressure, temperature and general observation of the patient. Normally, the nurse should remain with the patient for at least 5–10 minutes after a unit has been started to ensure any unexpected reaction is monitored (Torrance & Serginson 1999). Record carefully his intake of blood, any additional fluid given and his urine output. Check for any increase in pulse rate (tachycardia), lowering of his blood pressure (hypotension), any allergic response such as a sudden rash and, most importantly, any increase in temperature, or shivering and rigors. All these could indicate a reaction to the blood but symptoms such as increased pulse rate and lower blood pressure could also indicate further blood loss.

Continued

Table 2.1 Signs and symptoms associated with fluid and electrolyte problems—cont'd

Fluid and electrolyte intake	What could happen and your observations of the effect of this on a fluid balance chart as well as personal observation of the patient
A patient has returned from theatre and has had 2 litres of fluid over 24 hours, has not yet started to take fluids orally and has only passed 200 ml of urine in 24 hours.	Having a reduced urinary output is not uncommon in postoperative surgical patients (Torrance & Serginson 1999). This patient is experiencing what is known as low urine output or oliguria, as the flow of urine is less than 400 ml in 24 hours. Careful monitoring of his urine output on an hourly basis may be necessary.
A 60-year-old man has had major abdominal surgery. He has progressed to being allowed to eat as well as drink but he is reluctant to do either and his wound is not healing as well as anticipated.	It is important to encourage him to eat and drink as there is a correlation between good nutrition and wound healing. It is important to explain this to the patient and also find out why he is reluctant to eat and drink after his surgery. He may have fears about his wound bursting due to eating too much or he may still be feeling nauseated due to the effects of the anaesthetic. Whatever the reason, close observation and reassurance are essential in order for his wound to heal properly and for him to have any fears allayed postoperatively.

surgery should be 'well nourished and able to cope with a short period of pre- and postoperative starvation' (Torrance & Serginson 1999:103) but, as seen in *The Essence of Care* (Department of Health 2001, NHS Modernisation Agency 2003) it is evident that malnutrition is a problem in hospitals.

The possible causes of malnutrition in a patient undergoing surgery can be seen in Box 2.2.

You may already have considered that Mrs Gold will need care in a number of areas:
• Mental wellbeing.
• Physical preparation for undergoing surgery.

Box 2.2 Causes of malnutrition in the surgical patient

■ An underlying disease process causing a reduction in food intake and/or increased nutrient losses.
■ The metabolic response to trauma/surgery.
■ Enforced periods of nil by mouth.
■ Reduced appetite: may be further affected by pain/nausea/depression/anxiety.
■ Unfamiliar/unappetising hospital food.

(From: Ord H, Baker M (2010) Nutrition and the surgical patient. In: Pudner R, Nursing the surgical patient. Baillière Tindall, Edinburgh)

Activity

Consider Case history 2.1 as an experience you may have in a specific adult nursing placement or an exposure to other fields of practice clinical placement.

Case history 2.1

Mrs Gold, aged 56 years, has been admitted to hospital for surgery. She has had ulcerative colitis for 20 years which has been progressively affecting her quality of life. She has been admitted to hospital on numerous occasions over this period of time for palliative treatment, medication changes and surgery. Her nutritional status has become compromised, she has lost weight and has become depressed because of this and the constant exacerbation of her condition.

Activity

What will you need to know to be able to care for Mrs Gold leading up to her surgery?

- Nutritional needs during the whole of the perioperative period.
- Pain management.
- Medication.

This is an example of the type of learning experiences you might plan with your mentor to meet the NMC Standard in Box 2.3.

Paper to read prior to placement:

Fletcher J (2009) Identifying patients at risk of malnutrition: nutrition screening and assessment. Gastrointestinal Nursing 7(5): 12–17.

Tip

Prior to any practice placement experience, it is very important that you find out about the kinds of learning experiences you are likely to have and the health problems of the patients you are likely to come across. This will enable you to plan your pre-placement reading and also consider the kind of clinical skills that you may encounter to add to your increasing levels of competence and confidence.

Box 2.3 Developing learning plans with your mentor

Domain: Nursing Practice and decision making (NMC 2010)

Generic Standard for Competence (for all fields of practice)

Nurses must demonstrate a knowledge and understanding of how lifestyle, diversity and socioeconomic factors can affect health and illness and public health priorities.

They must meet the needs of people of all ages who may have overlapping physical and mental health problems, such as children and young people with addiction problems, eating disorders; and learning disabilities; adults with depression, eating disorders, dementia and drug and alcohol abuse; and older people with dementia, restricted lifestyles due to disability, and long-term illness.

NMC 2010 Standards of Competence (NMC 2010)

Managing pain

It must not be assumed that all patients undergoing surgery will experience pain or that it is an expected outcome. However, for many patients, and again depending on the surgery that has taken place, a certain level of pain or discomfort may be anticipated. Kitcatt (2010:103) states that *'pain is a complex, multidimensional experience and it is unique to the patient experiencing it . . . It is also a warning sign that something is wrong'*. This applies to any patient and not just those undergoing surgery. It is important, therefore, to understand the principles underpinning pain and why patients experience it, as well as the mental and physical effects on an individual.

Paper to read prior to placement:

Eid T, Bucknall T (2008) Documenting and implementing evidence-based post-operative pain management in older patients with hip fractures. Journal of Orthopaedic Nursing 12(2):90–98.

Managing infection control

Infection control is an essential aspect of a nurse's role in any field of practice and none more so than in a perioperative environment, especially in the operating theatre (see Ch. 8). Handwashing, for example, will have been introduced early in your nursing course, and many of you will have undertaken either formative or summative assessment in a clinical simulation laboratory in this essential nursing practice. Handwashing should be a normal day-to-day activity for adults and children, with more and more environments now adopting good practice in infection-free areas and the use of special antibacterial gels. Hospitals, nursing homes and other areas now ensure that visitors are also included in their good practice, with many hospitals setting up 'hand protection' stations at key points in hospital corridors and outside wards. You may, as a student, be given your own small bottle of gel to place in your pocket for daily use. Students in certain placements, such as mental health, have to adopt other mechanisms for infection control and handwashing due to the risk to patient safety and possibe self-harm if patients obtain access to these types of gels.

Paper to read prior to placement:

Col M (2007) Infection control: worlds apart primary and secondary care. British Journal of Community Nursing 12(7):301–306.

✔ Tip

Make sure you are familiar with the infection control policies and practice of your placement. Check that you are confident in handwashing technique and that you are aware of the possible consequences of not adopting good handwashing techniques and practices. Most of you will have undertaking handwashing as a key skill to learn prior to your first placement and some of you will have been assessed in this practice as well.

All students are expected to meet the standards for Essential Skills in Infection Control (see NMC 2010 Essential Skills Cluster: Infection Prevention and Control 21, 22–26).

Activity

Consider the NMC Standard and Competency Statement in Box 2.4 which includes generic statements and those applied specifically to mental health field of practice.

1. How could you use what you know about infection control policy and practices to enable you to meet the generic outcomes for any field of practice?
2. If you are following a mental health pathway, how could this help you to achieve your field-specific competency while undertaking a mental health-specific placement?

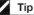 **Tip**

If undertaking the pathway to become a qualified mental health nurse, negotiating a short learning opportunity in a surgical placement could offer an insight into a client with mental health problems who has had a surgical procedure or intervention. Some of you will already have had this experience as part of a placement learning pathway (as described by the NMC [2010]) as good practice in developing a holistic view of client care.

Box 2.4 Domain 3: Nursing Practice and Decision Making (NMC 2010)

Generic standard for competence

All nurses must practise autonomously, compassionately, skilfully and safely, and must maintain dignity and promote health and wellbeing. They must assess and meet the full range of essential physical and mental health needs of people of all ages who come into their care. Where necessary, they must be able to provide safe and effective immediate care to all people prior to accessing or referring to specialist services irrespective of their field of practice. All nurses must also meet more complex and coexisting needs for people in their own nursing field of practice, in any setting including hospital, community and at home. All practice should be informed by the best available evidence and comply with local and national guidelines.

Decision making must be shared with service users, carers and families and informed by critical analysis of a full range of possible interventions, including the use of up-to-date technology. All nurses must also understand how behaviour, culture, socioeconomic and other factors, in the care environment and its location, can affect health, illness, health outcomes and public health priorities and take this into account in planning and delivering care.

Field standard for competence

Mental health nurses must draw on a range of evidence-based psychological, psychosocial and other complex therapeutic skills and interventions to provide person-centred support and care across all ages, in a way that supports self-determination and aids recovery. They must also promote improvements in physical and mental health and wellbeing and provide direct care to meet both the essential and complex physical and mental health needs of people with mental health problems.

Competencies

1. All nurses must use up-to-date knowledge and evidence to assess, plan, deliver and evaluate care, communicate findings, influence change and promote health and

Continued

Box 2.4 Domain 3: Nursing Practice and Decision Making (NMC 2010)—cont'd

best practice. They must make person-centred, evidence-based judgements and decisions, in partnership with others involved in the care process, to ensure high-quality care. They must be able to recognise when the complexity of clinical decisions requires specialist knowledge and expertise, and consult or refer accordingly.

1.1. Mental health nurses must be able to recognise and respond to the needs of all people who come into their care including babies, children and young people, pregnant and postnatal women, people with physical health problems, people with physical disabilities, people with learning disabilities, older people, and people with long-term problems such as cognitive impairment.

2. All nurses must possess a broad knowledge of the structure and function of the human body, and other relevant knowledge from the life, behavioural and social sciences as applied to health, ill health, disability, ageing and death. They must have an in-depth knowledge of common physical and mental health problems and treatments in their own field of practice, including co-morbidity and physiological and psychological vulnerability.

Cole (2007:24) explores some of the differences between infection control practice in primary and secondary care and examines the reasons for this.

Managing wounds and wound care

Surgical interventions lead to some kind of wound, whether it is a small incision as for a laparoscopy or insertion of an implant, or a major incision into the abdomen in order to reach major abdominal organs. They are usually made in 'a clean environment where asepsis is maintained at all times' (Pudner 2010).

Pudner (2010:51) states that the following are the 'main principles of surgical wound management':
- To achieve healing of the wound.
- To avoid complications, e.g. infection.
- To achieve good pain control.
- To ensure a cosmetically acceptable scar.

- To allow the individual to return to a normal lifestyle as soon as possible.

The kind of surgical placement you undertake will determine the experience you will gain in wound care and management, but these principles should be considered as a guide to determine learning experiences to obtain and skills to develop. Knowledge of wound healing, infection control and pain management are prerequisites for preparation for practice experience in a surgical placement (see Section 3 for integration of learning).

⟲ Activity

Read about the physiology of wound healing (surgical) and consider the factors that are essential for effective wound healing.

Re-visit the principles of asepsis and consider the key competences to achieve to meet the Essential Skills

Cluster on Infection Control (see NMC 2010 Essential Skills Cluster: Infection Prevention and Control 21, 22–26).

Revise and re-visit your handwashing skills prior to placement and find out what kind of policy is in place with regards to use of antibacterial hand gel.

Paper to read prior to placement:

Dowsett C (2002) The management of surgical wounds in a community setting. British Journal of Community Nursing 7(6 Suppl):33–38.

Managing stress and anxiety

Being anxious before undergoing a surgical procedure is a normal reaction for patients. However, there is research to show that although a certain level of anxiety is to be expected, higher levels can have a more profound impact on a patient's wellbeing. For example, Pritchard (2009:417) states that *'Anxious patients, particularly post-operative patients, appear to suffer more pain and can become more distressed by the presence of wound drains or urinary catheters'* and that *'the role of nurses is to ensure that the patient is fully prepared for the normal post-operative care a surgical operation may entail'*.

Managing anxiety and alleviating possible stress is a major part of caring for patients who are to undergo surgery (see Chs 6 and 9). Given that in the future, a significant number of surgical procedures will be experienced as day surgery, identifying patients at risk and offering them the support they need in the short term will become an important aspect of learning in any kind of surgical placement. It might form the basis of one of your main goals to achieve, for example: *'To determine the evidence base for preoperative and postoperative anxiety and to offer support to a*

patient during the perioperative period with the supervision of my mentor' (see Ch. 4 for goal statements).

Paper to read prior to placement:

Grieve R J (2002) Day surgery preoperative anxiety reduction and coping strategies. British Journal of Nursing 11(10):670–678.

Managing possible altered body image

Bob Price's (1990) explanation and model of body image is an excellent way of examining the way in which we normally see ourselves. When undergoing surgery, that normal perception of ourselves may be altered. Price considers that body image is actually made up of three different concepts: body ideal, body reality and body presentation. In brief, body reality *'refers to our body as it really is – tall, short, fat, thin, spotty, sallow, coarse'* and *'it is not how we would like our body to look, nor whether we find it pleasant or disagreeable. It is the body as seen and measured as objectively as humanly possible'* (Price 1990:4).

Body ideal, on the other hand, is when the body reality *'is measured constantly against an ideal of what we think the body should look like and how it should act. This ideal is carried in our head and may be applied not only to our own body reality, but that of others near and dear to us'* (Price 1990:6).

Body presentation is then related to how we dress and adorn our bodies but also, most importantly, *'the way in which it might move and pose its limbs were it to come to life'* (Price 1990:10). It is how we present ourselves and our body appearance to the social world.

Consider minor surgery involving the insertion of two or three sutures. For most people, this would not necessarily be problematic. Imagine if those sutures were to be inserted into the facial skin of a photographic model whose work was dependent on having a 'flawless' appearance, would their response be the same as someone whose work was not dependent on this? It is easy to see how concerns about body image can also have an effect on anxiety levels pre- and postoperatively.

It is important to consider the impact that any surgical intervention may have on a person regardless of anticipated disfigurement resulting from it. Learning about this prior to placement will give you knowledge to be able to consider a patient's needs during their perioperative care and also demonstrate your awareness of the links between physical aspects of care and social and psychological aspects.

Paper to read prior to placement:

Noone P (2010) Pre- and postoperative steps to improve body image following stoma surgery. Gastrointestinal Nursing 8(2):34–39.

References

Brogden, B.J., 2004. Clinical skills: importance of nutrition for acutely ill hospital patients. British Journal of Nursing 13 (15), 914–920.

Department of Health, 2001. The essence of care: patient-focused benchmarking for healthcare practitioners. DH, London.

Edwards, S.L., 1998. Malnutrition in hospital patients: where does it come from? British Journal of Nursing 7 (16), 971–974.

Fisher, A., McMillan, R., 2004. Integrated care pathways for day surgery patients. British Association of Day Surgery, London. Online. Available at: http://www.daysurgeryuk.net/bads/joomla/files/Handbooks/IntegratedCarePathways.pdf (accessed September 2011).

Gobbi, M., Cowen, M., Ugboma, D., 2006. Fluid and electrolyte balance. In:

Alexander, M., Fawcett, J.N., Runciman, P.J. (Eds.), Nursing practice hospital and home: the adult. Churchill Livingstone, Edinburgh: 763–785.

Holland, K., Jenkins, J., Solomon, J., Whittam, S. (Eds.), 2008. Applying the Roper–Logan–Tierney model in practice, 2nd ed. Churchill Livingstone, Edinburgh.

Kindlen, S., 2003. Physiology for health care and nursing. Churchill Livingstone, Edinburgh.

Kitcatt, S., 2010. Concepts of pain and the surgical patient. In: Pudner, R. (Ed.), Nursing the surgical patient, 3rd ed. Baillière Tindall, Edinburgh: 103–123.

NHS Modernisation Agency, 2003. Essence of care; patient-focused benchmarks for clinical governance. NHS, London.

Nursing and Midwifery Council, 2008. The code: standards of conduct, performance and ethics for nurses and midwives. NMC, London.

Nursing and Midwifery Council, 2010. Standards for pre-registration nursing education. Online. Available at: http://standards.nmc-uk.org/PreRegNursing/statutory/background/Pages/introduction.aspx (accessed May 2011).

Price, B., 1990. Body image – nursing concepts and care. Prentice Hall, London.

Pritchard, M.J., 2009. Managing anxiety in the elective surgical patient. British Journal of Nursing 18 (7), 416–419.

Pudner, R., 2010. Wound healing in the surgical patient. In: Pudner, R. (Ed.), Nursing the surgical patient. Baillière Tindall, Edinburgh: 51–76.

Roper, N., Logan, W., Tierney, A.J., 2000. The Roper, Logan and Tierney model of nursing – based on activities of living. Churchill Livingstone, Edinburgh.

Torrance, C., Serginson, E., 1999. Surgical nursing, 12th ed. Baillière Tindall/Royal College of Nursing, London.

Walker, J.A., 2002. Emotional and psychological preoperative preparation in adults. British Journal of Nursing 11 (8), 567–575.

Further reading

Black, P., 2009. Cultural and religious beliefs in stoma care nursing. British Journal of Nursing 18 (13), 790–793.

Brooker, C., Nicholl, M., 2011. Alexander's nursing practice, 4th ed. Churchill Livingstone, Edinburgh.

Burch, J., 2005. The pre- and postoperative nursing care for patients with a stoma. British Journal of Nursing 14 (6), 310–318.

Websites

The Breast Cancer Care UK website has some excellent resources on topics such as body image, surgical intervention and post-surgical expectations. There are also some excellent audio and video clips of women talking about their experiences: http://www.breastcancercare.org.uk/breast-cancer-breast-health/treatment-side-effects/surgery/ (accessed December 2011).

These links takes you to many different pages where you can discover not only patient stories of their experiences (http://www.nhs.uk/Planners/Yourhealth/Pages/Realstories.aspx) but also explanations of different kinds of surgical interventions such as removal of cataracts (http://www.nhs.uk/Search/Pages/Results.aspx?___JSSniffer=true&q=Cataract+surgery) and bowel cancer (http://www.nhs.uk/conditions/cancer-of-the-colon-rectum-or-bowel/pages/realsstoriesbowelcancer.aspx) (accessed December 2011).

3

Types of surgical nursing opportunities and clinical placements

CHAPTER AIMS

- To consider what a surgical placement is and what the environment might look like
- To determine the kind of learning opportunities a student might find in a surgical nursing placement
- To explore the various types of placements and the specific learning experiences to be gained

Surgical nursing placements

For many of you, a surgical nursing placement will be one of many placements you will experience in your programme of study, depending of course on the learning outcomes to be achieved as well as the specific requirements of your field of practice. In the main, placements where you are assessed in relation to the NMC Standards must be a minimum of 4 continuous weeks, but you may have shorter experiences in a surgical environment as part of a 'hub and spoke' approach to learning. Other terms used by the NMC (NMC 2010) are 'placement learning pathways', 'placement learning opportunities' and 'insight days', all focused on offering students opportunities to develop their skills and enhance their knowledge of 'understanding and supporting the patient journey' (NMC 2010:40).

The length of time in a placement will be determined initially by your curriculum requirements. Discussion with your mentor about what you can realistically achieve in terms of clinical skills and patient care experience will ensure you meet the required learning outcomes and competences for that placement (see Ch. 4 for a discussion of placement learning opportunities).

⟐ Activity

Imagine you have been told that your next placement is a surgical nursing one and you have no prior experience of visiting one nor have you worked on one as a healthcare assistant.

What do you imagine the environment will look like that is different to a medical nursing placement? Consider the explanations offered in Chapters 1 and 2 regarding the nature of surgical nursing and section on Description of a Surgical ward for further discussion of what a surgical ward may look like.

Continued

In the main, placements identified as 'surgical' are normally named or relate to various aspects of medical care or anatomy and physiology/systems of the body. Each one is a specialty with specific nursing-related care, but each involves the same perioperative process. Here are some examples:

- Orthopaedic surgery.
- Ear, nose and throat surgery.
- Gynaecology surgery.
- Vascular surgery.
- Abdominal surgery.
- Renal and urinary tract surgery.
- Neurological surgery.
- Ophthalmic surgery.
- Thoracic/chest surgery.
- Breast surgery.
- Cardiac surgery.
- Plastic surgery.

Consider all these types of surgery and find out what 'body systems' they are associated with. Use a nursing dictionary to help you identify the kind of surgery that normally takes place in your placement.

You will have discovered the following:
- Orthopaedic surgery involves surgery of the musculoskeletal system.
- Ear, nose and throat surgery involves surgery of the ear, nose and throat, including the larynx.
- Gynaecology surgery involves surgery of the female reproductive system.
- Vascular surgery involves surgery of the arteries and veins.
- Abdominal surgery involves surgery of abdominal organs such as liver, bowel, stomach, gall bladder.
- Renal and urinary tract surgery involves surgery of the kidney and related organs and systems.
- Neurological surgery involves surgery of the brain and spinal cord.
- Ophthalmic surgery involves surgery of the eye and related structures.
- Thoracic/chest surgery involves surgery of the respiratory organs.
- Breast surgery involves surgery of the breast – male and female.
- Cardiac surgery involves surgery of the heart.
- Plastic surgery involves reconstructive surgery in varied parts of the body.

You may be undertaking a placement that is simply identified as a general surgical ward, and here you may meet patients undergoing a range of surgical interventions. It is up to you to be knowledgable about general and specific surgery, as well as anatomy and physiology. (We explore why it is important to revise anatomy and physiology prior to your placement throughout the book, but especially in Section 3.)

Further reading related to surgical placements can be found at the end of Chapter 4.

Description of a surgical ward

It is important to remember that each hospital and its layout varies. All we can consider here is a basic idea of what a surgical ward might look like and the kind of equipment and activities you are likely to encounter.

A surgical ward is usually a very busy environment, with patients being taken back and forth to theatre by nurses, theatre attendants and other relevant personnel. (Other linked placements are described in Section 2: for example, the operating theatre.)

Activity

Consider what you imagine a surgical ward might look like. Have a look at some photos on the Internet or in books to compare current images and past images.

If you have been a patient or visitor on a surgical ward, is your first impression of the placement the same as you recall?

When you go to the placement for the first time, note the layout of the ward and what makes it identifiable as a surgical placement as opposed to an outpatient placement. What kinds of objects and activities make it identifiable as such?

Read Holland's (1993) article, which describes an ethnographic study carried out on a surgical ward, for a description of what she calls 'cultural artefacts' and specific practices she observed which clearly identified it as a surgical ward. Specific language used in communication between nurses was also an indicator. (See Box 3.1 for some of her observations.)

Box 3.1 Data from an ethnographic description of a nursing cultural scene

Description of the ward

The patients who were part of this particular cultural scene were allowed in on the basis that they had a medically diagnosed, specific, disordered body function which required surgical intervention. The nature of their treatment gave the ward its name (i.e. a surgical ward), thus differentiating it from others within the hospital.

For instance, domain analysis of 'kinds of surgical intervention' – right inguinal hernia repair, mid-thigh amputation, appendicectomy, draining of rectal abscess, transurethral prostatectomy.

Description by one nurse of what would make them take someone's temperature or not

Um well, the charts, really I know I shouldn't say that but I go to the charts... If someone is pre-op, it should be morning and evening... post-op should be 4-hourly for signs of infection and until the wound heals sufficiently... If they look like they've got a temperature or feel hot, take it in-between times, if they were chesty or look like they've got a urine infection... (Mary)

(From Holland 1993)

Some students, however, are not happy about where they are to undertake their placement, complaining that they won't learning anything there. This is often an issue of perception, perhaps influenced through personal experience or that of a relative.

⟨⟩ Reflection point

Consider the following example from a student at the beginning of their second year of study.

'I am going to a day surgery ward. What am I going to learn there? I want to be caring for patients who have big operations and lots going on. It's going to be really repetitive and boring.'

We [KH and Student] discussed generally the kinds of experience he could have and he was advised to set very clear learning goals with regards to the patient journey.

On his return from placement, he said he had had a brilliant time and had learned loads of things! Among these, he had experienced meeting a patient, going with him to theatre, staying with him during surgery, staying with him in the recovery room and being there for him when he woke up in a strange environment and then taking him back to the ward and caring for him until he was discharged home from hospital that evening.

It had not been possible for the student to follow up the patient after his discharge home, but this is one aspect of care that can be negotiated with your mentor. It may be possible to visit patients in their home/community setting through liaising with the health centre/district nurse who may be in charge of their care.

✓ Tip

Consider how your placement experience might help you to attain the NMC competences. For those of you who are expected to meet the NMC 2004 Standards and Competencies, the wording of those identified here will be similar – please note, however, that there are now field-specific competencies to achieve. See Box 3.2 for an example for adult students undertaking the adult nursing pathway.

Box 3.2 Domain: Nursing Practice and Decision Making (NMC 2010)

Generic Standard for Competence

Graduate nurses must practise in a compassionate, respectful way, maintaining the dignity and wellbeing of all concerned. Decision making must be person-focused, and through a process of critical analysis leading to a range of technical skills and nursing interventions from basic to highly complex. They must practise in a safe and confident manner, in various care settings, understanding how the environment and location of care delivery can have an impact on health and outcomes. All practice must be based on current evidence and up-to-date technology.

Box 3.2 Domain: Nursing Practice and Decision Making (NMC 2010)—cont'd

Competencies

1. *All nurses must work closely with individuals, groups and carers, using a range of skills to carry out comprehensive, systematic and holistic assessments. These must take into account current and previous physical, social, cultural, psychological, spiritual, genetic and environmental factors that may be relevant to the individuals and their families.*

   1.1. *Adult nurses must safely use a range of diagnostic and clinical skills, complemented by existing and developing technology, to assess the nursing care of individuals undergoing therapeutic or clinical interventions.*

2. *All nurses must listen, recognise and respond to an individual's physical, social and psychological needs. They must then plan, deliver and evaluate technically safe, competent, person-centred care that addresses all their daily activities, in partnership with people and their carers, families and other professionals.*

   2.1. *Adult nurses must safely use invasive and non-invasive procedures, technological support and pharmacological management for medical and surgical nursing practice. They must take account of individual needs and preferences as well as any existing or long-term health problems.*

Placement learning opportunities and pathways in surgical nursing placements

The NMC (2010) guidance stresses the importance of placement learning in the community and hospital in order to gain a holistic understanding of patients' journeys through health and social care services as well as the competencies to be able to work on registration in either environment. As a student whose main placement is on a surgical ward, how then can you gain experience in the community?

Consider the following pathway options which include various learning opportunities and experiences.

Mapping of potential surgical placement learning pathways

Example for a 10-week placement: the patient journey (pre-planned pathway) In this option, you can see that as a 'pre-planned' pathway, the student experience has been mapped out for a hospital placement with a clearly defined journey.

10-week Placement: the patient journey (pre-planned pathway)			
Placement 1	**Placement 2**	**Placement 3**	**Placement 4**
Orthopaedic ward (4 weeks)	Operating theatre (1 week)	Postoperative recovery (1 week)	Orthopaedic ward (4 weeks)

Some of you will already have experienced this kind of planned surgical experience.

Example for an 8-week placement: the patient experience and interprofessional working (learning outcomes negotiated with mentor and personal tutor) In this option, however, there are still experiences which enable the student to gain an understanding of what a patient's surgical journey may be like, but this pattern is a negotiated learning experience which many of you know as a 'hub and spoke' model, or a 'base and insight learning days' approach. In this kind of experience, the interprofessional aspects can be much more clearly defined and if you have to gain this experience to meet specific learning outcomes on interprofessional working in practice, then this negotiated learning would be beneficial. It is important to remember that in any kind of placement learning pathway, negotiating learning outcomes around interprofessional working is an essential part of achieving your NMC competences to practice.

Example for a 14-week placement: an integrated hospital/community plan: the patient experience and journey (a pre-planned allocation pathway) This option is a pre-planned and allocated one, usually by the placement learning unit at university, in collaboration with practice colleagues such as practice education facilitators.

This is the kind of placement that a student may undertake in the final year of their programme of study, when they would be assessed as fit for practice by their sign off

8-week Placement: the patient experience and interprofessional working

Placement 1	Day 1	Day 2	Day 3	Day 4	Day 5/6
Orthopaedic ward (8 weeks with specialist days negotiated over the 8 weeks)	Outpatients clinic/arthroplasty surgery	Rehabilitatation; physiotherapy unit	Rehabilitation: occupational therapist	Theatre: total hip replacement surgery	2 days in trauma: accident and emergency

14-week Placement: an integrated hospital and community plan – the patient experience and journey

Placement 1	Placement 2	Placement 3	Placement 4
Community health centre: case load and caring for a patient following orthopaedic surgery (5 weeks)	Orthopaedic ward: care of patients following surgery (2 weeks)	Operating theatre: orthopaedic surgery (1 week)	Community health centre (6 weeks)

Activity

Imagine you have an 8-week allocation to a surgical placement, a ward that specialises in cardiothoracic surgery. What kind of surgery would patients experience on this ward?

Plan a learning experience you would like to gain during the 8 weeks, taking account of all resources available. You will find many of these in Chapter 4 regarding university and placement information, and throughout the book with regards to possible learning outcomes and surgical interventions. Use these and any others discussed with your personal tutor to negotiate learning with your named mentor and the practice team.

---

mentor. Importantly, however, there is the option and opportunity within their allocated case load to gain leadership and management competencies as well as those of communication and interpersonal skills, nursing practice and decision making and professional values, but including a 'surgical' patient journey.

Note: the NMC has stated that 4 weeks is the minimum number of weeks for a student to be assessed in a clinical placement with regards to their competences. All of these placement options reflect this.

Summary

As well as focusing learning to prepare yourself for specific surgical nursing placements, there is a need to focus on general expectations in relation to what you are expected to achieve by your university as well as the specific programme of study you are undertaking. Chapter 4 considers these in more detail.

References

Holland, C.K., 1993. An ethnographic study of nursing culture as an exploration for determining the existence of a system of ritual. Journal of Advanced Nursing 18, 1461–1470.

Nursing and Midwifery Council, 2010. Standards for pre-registration nursing education. NMC, London. Online. Available at: http://standards.nmc-uk.org/PreRegNursing/statutory/background/Pages/introduction.aspx (accessed September 2011).

Further reading

Callaghan, A., 2010. Student nurses' perceptions of learning in a perioperative placement. Journal of Advanced Nursing 67 (4), 854–864.

Callaghan, P., 2007. Rethinking clinical placements for mental health nursing students. Mental Health Practice 10 (5), 18–20.

Hughes, S., 2006. Evaluating operating theatre experience. Journal of Perioperative Practice 16 (6), 290–298.

Sampson, H., 2006. Introducing student nurses to operating department nursing. Journal of Perioperative Practice 16 (2), 87–94.

Website

RCN website for student nurses and clinical placement experiences with a range of other resources for student nurses: http://nursingstandard.rcnpublishing.co.uk/students/clinical-placements/placement-advice/picking-the-right-placement/student-nurses-should-vary-their-placements (accessed December 2011).

4

Preparation for learning in practice

CHAPTER AIMS

- To introduce the principles of learning in practice
- To identify teachers who will be involved in supervision, teaching and assessing in practice and at university
- To identify what to consider pre-placement
- To consider how to meet some of the NMC Standards and Competencies during the placement experience

Introduction

Levett-Jones and Bourgeois (2009) outline much of what we discuss in this section and others, and they offer excellent advice and guidance for students prior to, during and after placements. If you are reading this book, you will probably be undertaking either a programme of study where the course is clearly divided into a 1-year common foundation programme (CFP) and a 2-year branch programme (NMC 2004) or one where there is no CFP and branch evident but still requires a programme of study which enables you to achieve outcomes (NMC 2010a) which are field of practice specific (what was branch outcomes).

Regardless of which NMC outcomes you are having to achieve, the principles remain the same. You must also ensure that you adhere to both the student. Guidance on Professional Conduct (NMC 2009) and your future Code: Standards of Conduct, Performance and Ethics for Nurses and Midwives (NMC 2008). It is very important that you read these and discuss them with your personal tutor before undertaking placement learning and also your mentor when you meet for the first time.

Each university will have its own curriculum expectations with regards to achievement of learning outcomes and assignment requirements, but every student, through whatever practice assessment documents and processes developed, has to achieve the NMC Standards and Competencies in theory and practice in order to become a registered nurse. These combined requirements lead to an academic award (in future, a degree will be the minimum academic award to enter the nursing profession) and a professional award and subsequent registration as a nurse (RN).

To help you achieve these in a clinical placement context, you will be supported by a named mentor and a number of other qualified nurses (now known as registrants) as well as other healthcare workers and professionals. We have already considered the general roles of some of these in Chapter 1, but it is important for you to consider the specific roles and responsibilities of those who will facilitate your learning and be responsible for assessing your knowledge and skills in a placement.

Key roles linked to student learning in practice

The mentor

Every student who is to gain a clinical placement learning experience has to have a named mentor (mandatory requirement of the NMC (2008)) who will be their main facilitator of learning, their supervisor and the assessor of their practice. All mentors should be experienced nurses who have completed a course of mentorship preparation or have an equivalent qualification in their own field which is recognised as being appropriate to supervise and assess student nurses in practice. (This latter individual will only be able to undertake this role in specific placements and not at the major progression points in the new NMC (2010a) guidance for curriculum delivery.) It is the mentor who is responsible for assessing your learning and competence in practice. As well as your practice assessment document, the mentor will also complete your ongoing record of achievement (ORA) (NMC 2007). (See Box 4.1 for an example of the mentor role and expectations of you as a student in relation to the ORA. Please note that this is only a very brief version for illustration purposes and that all universities will have different and very detailed practice assessment documentation.)

Your main mentor will be supported in their role by a number of other appropriate personnel and, in some placements, more senior student nurses will take an active role in the teaching and support of students as part of their role in transition learning outcomes.

Box 4.1 Example of possible guidance notes for students and mentors during a placement

The assessment process

Week 1

- Student MUST negotiate with their mentor a time for their initial interview to discuss learning needs and goals and agree an action plan for achievement.
- Student MUST share with their mentor their ongoing record of achievement from any previous placements and any action plans resulting from their last assessment of learning in practice.
- Student will ensure that mentors are aware of any non-practice assessments they need to complete which may require their support for achieving, such as a client-focused assessment or evidence-based practice on a placement-specific topic.
- Student may also have additional practice-based assessments to achieve in the placement, such as medicine management, handwashing skills or (ward/patient care) management.

Box 4.1 Example of possible guidance notes for students and mentors during a placement—cont'd

Mid-point placement experience

■ Student and mentor will ensure that they meet to discuss progress at some point halfway through their placement experience and also to determine if any actions from previous placement (ORA information) are being achieved. Evidence of progress will be gathered from a range of sources, including student skills record/practice assessment documents, other qualified nursing staff (registrants) and other health workers in direct contact on a regular basis with the student.

■ Student MUST receive constructive feedback from their mentor at this point and also on an ongoing basis. Their mentor must ensure that the student is being taught new skills and gaining new knowledge through ongoing evaluation of learning and any deficit from their original agreed action plan can be re-negotiated if required. This mid-point meeting is an essential one for the student who may require additional support from their mentor to achieve successful completion of their practice assessment in this placement.

Final placement period

■ Student and mentor MUST meet during the final week of placement and a suitable time agreed. (The importance of this final placement assessment is critical for those students in their final placement as their practice will be required to be assessed by the sign off mentor.) All evidence must be available about their progress on the placement and all documents available for discussion and signatures. Self-evaluation may be required as part of their practice assessment documents.

■ It is at this stage that the student has to offer clear evidence that they have achieved their goals, met the required NMC competencies for the placement and a record made of their overall performance during their placement.

■ Ongoing record of practice assessment could indicate decisions by the mentor such as:

■ *Achieved*: all outcomes achieved competently, safely and professional behaviour appropriate.

■ *Not achieved*: although some outcomes achieved, the student's overall performance has not met the required standard or achieved required NMC competencies for this placement.

■ Student and mentor discuss the outcomes and agree subsequent actions according to university policies.

> ✓ **Tip**
>
> If you are a senior student undertaking a surgical placement in your final year of study, it is an ideal opportunity not only to learn to care for patients and their families in this environment but also to help less experienced students learn how to care for a patient undergoing surgery.
>
> Agree a learning goal with your mentor to do this and don't forget, make it **SMART:** **S**pecific, **M**easurable, **A**chievable, **R**ealistic and **T**imely (Fowler 1998). For example, to teach a first year student nurse how to prepare a patient for surgery:
>
> - **S**pecific: focuses on a very specific topic.
> - **M**easurable: it can be tested by questions and answers and by how the student prepares a patient for surgery.
> - **A**chievable: this is a surgical ward with patients going to operating theatre every day of the week.
> - **R**ealistic: maybe you have had a lecture and participated in a seminar at university about teaching others, and this is also your second surgical placement in 3 years so you have more than a basic knowledge of what is required.
> - **T**imely: it can be achieved in the student's placement experience regardless of length and you will be able to see the impact of your teaching.
>
> Setting goals like this with your mentor not only demonstrates your willingness to learn but also helps you to expand your own knowledge and skills and consolidate previous learning.

> 🔊 **Activity**
>
> In preparation for meeting your mentor, check out any online information you can access about your surgical placement, as well as the hospital or other environment where it will be. Check out the kind of surgery that takes place there and write out a draft plan of what you want to experience and learn during the time you are there. This could be a short placement within a larger placement learning pathway (or a 'hub and spoke' placement) or a single placement where there may be opportunities to experience a snapshot of a total patient experience.

Sign off mentor

The role of the sign off mentor is to 'sign off' a student's proficiency in the NMC Standards and Competencies at the end of their NMC-approved programme (Levett-Jones & Bourgeois 2009). This role is undertaken in the final placement only, but the decision will be based on the decisions of other mentors who have recorded and approved the student's progress in their ongoing record of achievement in previous placements. These mentors are critical to the assessment of a student's fitness to practice as a safe and effective qualified nurse, and they are responsible and accountable for providing the evidence on which the sign off mentor makes their final assessment. To be a sign off mentor, the qualified nurse must have undertaken a further course beyond that of mentorship.

As a student in your final placement, it is essential that you meet with the sign off mentor for the equivalent of 1 hour per week, in addition to the 40% of time working with your mentor normally. This is to ensure ongoing and constructive feedback is given as to your progress in the placement, and also builds on your previous ongoing record of achievement. (Please refer to the full NMC guidance on issues of confidentiality and access to your ongoing record of achievement at: http://www.nmc-uk.org/Documents/Circulars/2007circulars/NMC%20circular%2033_2007.pdf.)

Practice education facilitator

This is a relatively new role in practice education. Practice education facilitators (PEFs) are mainly employed to support mentors in their role and to act as a link between them and colleagues in universities. A study by Carlisle et al (2009:715), evaluating the role in Scotland, found that:

> *Findings indicate that the PEF role has been accepted widely across Scotland and is seen as valuable to the development of quality clinical learning environments. PEFs provide support and guidance for mentors when dealing with 'failing' students, and encourage the identification of innovative learning opportunities. PEFs play an active part in student evaluation of their placements, but further work is needed in order that the feedback to clinical areas and mentors is timely.*

Some PEFs will work with mentors to develop supplementary learning opportunities for students in practice, such as study days, workshops and shared learning opportunities with other healthcare professionals.

PEFs also work with mentors and link teachers/tutors from universities, to develop and ensure that student placements are quality learning environments. They will also be involved in evaluation of your learning experience in the placement and the educational audit, whereby a specific tool is used by the placement area to evaluate the quality of the overall learning environment, to which you will also have contributed.

Link teacher

The link teacher role was introduced to ensure that there remained strong links between education and service areas when nursing education was transferred into the higher education sector in the UK. Initially, this role was key to the successful development of the learning environment in clinical practice, working with ward managers and mentors to develop placement learning opportunities and experiences for students as well as ensuring their quality. Of late, this role has become less visible but the link teacher still has a key role to play in ensuring that the areas which they link with support student learning (Arkell & Bayliss; Pratt 2007). You can check the identity of your placement link tutor through the placement learning information on your university website and also when you arrive in your allocated placement.

> ✔ **Tip**
>
> It is important to make a note of your link teacher's name in your student diary because there may be a time when you need to contact the university directly, for example to speak with your personal tutor who may not be available, and the placement link teacher may be able to help you instead.

In many areas, the link teacher works closely with the PEFs in ensuring good learning experiences for students, and some still retain hands-on clinical care and case loads. Some are also employed as lecturer–practitioners by NHS organisations, where they work half-time in the university and half-time in a clinical specialty (Buchan et al 2008).

Key preparation before starting your placement

Roberts (2010) outlines key things that you can do to prepare before starting a clinical placement. These include making sure you attend your planned clinical skills and simulated learning sessions and, if an opportunity is planned into the timetable, undertake some additional practice in the clinical skills classroom, either on your own or with a colleague, ensuring that your skills tutors are aware that you are doing so.

Practising skills prior to undertaking a placement can enhance your confidence when asked to undertake tasks. Taking a blood pressure, for example, is an essential skill to learn if undertaking a surgical placement, given the importance of blood pressure as an indicator of potential problems post-surgery such as shock due to excessive loss of blood.

Some universities have excellent resources for students to use on their student learning sites, accessible via personal passwords. You can also find useful resources and books which make a valued addition to pre-placement preparation (for example, see: http://www.oup.com/uk/orc/bin/9780199534456/01student/checklists/ (accessed December 2011)).

Activity

Log on to your university learning resource centre (such as BlackBoard) and find the online learning material with regards to clinical skills or preparation for practice placements. (See the University of Nottingham for an example of practice learning pages: http://www.nottingham.ac.uk/nursing/practice-learning/index.aspx (accessed December 2011).)

Tip

Use the following as a checklist prior to starting your placement.

Item	Yes	No
Checked dates of placement		
Found out where it is		
Found out best way to get there		
What time to arrive		
What to take with me		
What to wear (see uniform options)		
Name of mentor and ward/unit/health centre manager/sister		
Logged on to the course learning resource centre (Intranet/password needed) and checked for any messages from programme/module leader/personal tutor		
Found out information available on any practice learning links on the school website		

Continued

✅ Tip—cont'd

Found out link teacher's name for the placement		
Undertaken some initial reading about the kinds of patient problems I may come across and the possible care of the patients		
Obtained a personal file for using at home to make notes on various health problems, signs and symptoms, medications, surgical interventions, etc.		
If time, practice some skills relevant to placement in clinical skills lab with teacher agreement		
Refresh knowledge in any notes undertaken in lectures/seminars at university		
Obtain at least one book from library or other resource which is relevant to the clinical placement, e.g. Pudner (2010)		
Ensure plenty of time to get to placement on the first day		

✅ Tip

Make sure you visit your placement whenever possible prior to commencing your actual clinical experience and obtain the name of your mentor and the first week's off duty (the hours of learning practice noted on the nursing duty rota, usually posted on the staff notice board) which may also be negotiated with your mentor when you get there.

Key university roles and professional conduct issues and practices in ensuring successful learning outcomes and opportunities in clinical placements

The personal tutor

The role of the personal tutor is central to the successful transition and journey through your specific field of practice (branch) pathway and programme of study.

It is expected that all students are allocated a personal tutor, normally from their own field of practice such as mental health, learning disability, adult or children and young people's nursing. A study by Por and Barriball (2008:100) showed that lecturers who undertook this role provided a range of activities from the *'provision of pastoral care and acting as a referral agent to other services such as student support networks, to monitoring student progress and giving academic support when required'*. The main types of support that most students required were linked to these issues.

Activity

Discuss with your personal tutor what they consider their role to be and how you can ensure that both of you can work together with regards to achieving your outcomes during clinical placement.

Many universities have specific criteria for the role and also guidance for what students expect from personal tutors and vice versa. Find out if your

Continued

university has a document of this kind and discuss it with your personal tutor when meeting for the first time.

Your personal tutor will play a key role in helping you to achieve your personal and professional development goals or similar processes, which involves discussion of overall progress on your programme (including placement learning) as well as keeping records of achievements in a portfolio (Timmins 2008).

Expectations of being a student in practice placement

During your clinical placement, you will be a supernumerary member of the team. It is important to understand what this does and does not mean. Being supernumerary means that even though your name might appear on the staff duty rota, you are not counted in the staff numbers as being a member of the workforce on that shift.

Supernumerary does not mean that you do not become involved in *learning to work* alongside your mentor and other members of staff and telling staff in the placement that you cannot do something because you are there only to observe. It also does not mean that you can come and go as you please (you may think this is extreme and wouldn't happen – trust us, it has been known!), unless of course you have come to an arrangement with your mentor in the placement regarding specific learning hours. Some placements, for example outpatient departments, only open 8 am to 5 pm Monday to Friday; if that is the case then you also work, or a better word is 'practice', within those hours as required by the university. Some of you might also be on placement for 3 days a week and then at university for the other 2 days. (See Roberts (2010) for an explanation of some of the issues with regards to supernumerary status (see Box 4.2).)

Box 4.2 Excerpt from Roberts (2010) on supernumerary status and its importance

'Your role as a learner in practice is strengthened by "supernumerary status". As a student nurse you do not "go to work" in the way that the professionals and other paid staff do. You go to a placement to "learn" for a short time and then move to another placement to learn more. In your placement you are of course working as well (e.g. assisting patients, learning nursing procedures, attending case conferences, etc.) but as a student nurse you are there principally to learn through the work you are doing' (Roberts 2010:138).

Expected professional conduct and behaviour: fitness to practice

In 2009, the NMC published its first edition Guidance on Professional Conduct for Nursing and Midwifery Students and a second edition with minor amendments was published in September 2010. This new guidance is a very important document for all students regardless of the individual programme of study requirements or practice placement, and as such its implications for students must be stressed. You can read it in full at: http://www.nmc-uk.org/Students/Guidance-for-students/ (accessed December 2011).

In addition, another critically important document for students is the guidance on good health and good character (NMC 2010b) which can be read in full at: http://www.nmc-uk.org/Students/Good-Health-and-Good-Character-for-students-nurses-and-midwives/ (accessed December 2011).

So what do these mean for you as a student going into a clinical placement? In brief, good health (and poor health) and good character are defined as follows (NMC 2010b):

Good character

1. Good character is important and is central to the code in that nurses and midwives must be honest and trustworthy. Good character is based on an individual's conduct, behaviour and attitude. It also takes account of any convictions, cautions and pending charges that are likely to be incompatible with professional registration. A person's character must be sufficiently good for them to be capable of safe and effective practice without supervision.

Good health

2. Good health is necessary to undertake practice as a nurse or midwife. Good health means that a person must be capable of safe and effective practice without supervision. It does not mean the absence of any disability or health condition. Many disabled people and those with health conditions are able to practise with or without adjustments to support their practice.

Poor health

3. If a nurse or midwife is in poor health it means that they are affected by a physical or mental health condition that impairs their ability to practice without supervision.
4. Applicants who declare health conditions or disabilities should be assessed where appropriate with support from a disability services team or adviser. Any assessment should focus on what reasonable adjustments can be made to support the applicant to achieve entry to or maintenance on our register.

🔵 Activity

Read the meaning of these for students in the NMC Guidance on Professional Conduct (see Box 4.3) and consider their importance for undertaking a surgical placement. Also check out the NMC website for up-to-date information on professional practice and student-related issues: http://www.nmc-uk.org/ (accessed December 2011).

Box 4.3 Extract from the NMC (2009) *Guidance on Professional Conduct for Nursing and Midwifery Students*

What do good health, good character and fitness to practise mean?

The NMC provides guidance on good health, good character and fitness to practice.

Good health *is necessary to undertake practice as a nurse or a midwife. Good health means that a person must be capable of safe and effective practice without supervision. It does not mean the absence of any disability or health condition. Many disabled people and those with long-term health conditions are able to practise with or without adjustments to support their practice.*

Good character *is important as nurses and midwives must be honest and trustworthy. Good character is based on a person's conduct, behaviour and attitude. It also takes account of any convictions and cautions that are not considered to be compatible with professional registration and that might bring the profession into disrepute. A person's character must be sufficiently good for them to be capable of safe and effective practice without supervision.*

Continued

Box 4.3 Extract from the NMC (2009) *Guidance on Professional Conduct for Nursing and Midwifery Students* — cont'd

Fitness to practice *means having the skills, knowledge, good health and good character to do your job safely and effectively. Your **fitness to practice** as a student will be assessed throughout your pre-registration programme and, if there are ever concerns, these will be investigated and addressed by the university.*

*You should familiarise yourself with the student regulations and **fitness to practice** procedures in your university. Ask your tutor or mentor for more information*

Possible learning outcomes to be achieved in a surgical placement

To enable you to consider some possible learning goals to achieve in a surgical placement, we have identified one competency statement from each of the four NMC (2010) domains to illustrate how you can negotiate relevant experience and associated knowledge and skills to help you attain successful outcomes in these areas. Each one has an activity that you can use to help you prior to your surgical placement.

General learning outcomes (NMC Gereric Standards examples)

Domain: Professional Values

9. *All nurses must appreciate the value of evidence in practice, be able to understand and appraise research, apply relevant theory and research findings to their work and identify areas for further investigation.*

This is a competence which underpins the achievement of many other competencies and is an essential part of undertaking a qualified nurse's role (Holland & Rees 2010). How you approach this competence will depend very much on where you are in your programme of study prior to undertaking a surgical placement. If a first year student, you may just be beginning your journey of discovery with regards to what is evidence

for practice, how you find it and how to understand and evaluate it in order to be able to determine whether it is evidence that you can use in your practice or to support your assignment work (Holland 2010). However, this is a competence that you must achieve at some point in your programme of study to become a qualified nurse, and which your sign off mentor will expect to see evidence for at the end of your programme of study.

The following activity helps you to develop knowledge in preparation for your placement experience and also enhances your developing skills of searching for evidence, critiquing its relevance for practice and sharing it with other colleagues.

◆ Activity

Find three articles on one aspect of surgical care, which can include the whole perioperative period. (These can be related to one specific focus across all fields of practice or related to one specific field of practice.)

Summarise the evidence and present it to your fellow students at an appropriate opportunity in your placement and following discussion with your mentor.

Determine whether the findings of these research papers could help change practice in your placement and the care of patients.

To help you with this activity, here are some examples of papers you could use to support pre-placement learning and develop your critique skills on the subject of anxiety and surgery.

- Grieve R J (2002) Day surgery preoperative anxiety reduction and coping strategies. British Journal of Nursing 11(10):670–678.
- Stirling L (2006) Reduction and management of perioperative anxiety. British Journal of Nursing 15 (7):359–361.
- Pritchard M J (2009) Managing anxiety in the elective surgical patient. British Journal of Nursing 18(7):416–419.

Also, see Holland & Rees (2010) at: http://www.oup.com/uk/orc/bin/9780199563104/01student/chapters/ (accessed December 2011) for examples of article evaluation tools (Ch. 7) and other material regarding evidence-based practice resources.

You can also access the Foundation of Nursing Studies website where you will find a range of information about the impact on practice and practice development that some of their funded projects have made: http://www.fons.org/default.aspx (accessed December 2011).

Domain: Communication and Interpersonal Skills

2. All nurses must use a range of communication skills and technologies to support person-centred care and enhance quality and safety. They must ensure people receive all the information they need in a language and manner that allows them to make informed choices and share decision making. They must recognise when language interpretation or other communication support is needed and know how to obtain it.

During your placement experience, you will meet and care for patients and their families from a wide range of different cultures whose first language is not English, and where communication with carers may not always be easy for the patient or the carers. You will also meet other patients who have different kinds of communication needs, such as deafness or speech impediment. In other situations, you may also find patients who are unconscious for a prolonged period of time, for example during surgery or on intensive care units following surgery. How will you learn to identify communication needs when the patient is unable to articulate their fears and anxiety?

Looking at Case history 4.1, consider what your actions would be in the situation, and then set yourself a learning goal to meet this competency to discuss with your mentor.

Case history 4.1

On your first day on placement, you are asked by your mentor to stay with an elderly Polish man who will be going to theatre soon. You can see he still has his hearing aid in (Gilmour 2010, p.20) but when you introduce yourself to him and tell him you will be staying with him until it is time for him to go to the operating theatre for the operation on his leg (he is expected to be considered for an amputation), it is clear that he does not fully understand you and begins to ask why he is going to theatre for surgery on his leg and what is going to happen to him. When asked, he knows where he is, which hospital he is in, his name and what has happened to him so far to prepare him physically for going to theatre.

Relating this scenario to the competency, it is clear that managing this kind of situation effectively within your own sphere of experience and knowledge will enable you to achieve many of the different elements required:

- It is clear that the patient does not seem confused from the questions you have asked him based on your knowledge of how to find out if the patient is confused about his situation.

- It is also clear that he is able to hear you as he still has his hearing aid in and this can safely stay in until he is in the anaesthetic room to aid communication until he is anaesthetised (Gilmour 2010).
- He can obviously understand what you are saying in English as he has responded to your basic questions to try and determine if he has become confused for some reason.

So what could be wrong ?

The main problem appears to be around why he is going to theatre for surgery on his leg and what is going to happen to him. Given that he will be going to theatre soon, this is a situation which needs to be resolved urgently in order that he is reassured and so that he understands clearly what options were involved when he gave informed consent. It is important to ensure people receive all the information they need in a language and manner that allows them to make informed choices and share decision making.

It is essential to tell your mentor immediately. Reassure the patient that you will get someone to come and talk to him again about his surgery and that you will come back to sit with him. If it is agreeable to him, reassure him that you will go with him to the theatre environment.

The mentor, as a qualified nurse who is bound by the NMC Code, should immediately call the surgical team and ask one of them to come and explain again to the patient about his surgery and what is going to take place.

You can see from this possible scenario that being a nurse requires not only effective communication and good interpersonal skills but also a knowledge of ethical issues involved in decision making and informed consent, and consideration of all the possible options regarding the questions of patients.

A goal from this learning exercise could be that you will: *consider all aspects of communication when patients are admitted to hospital, with a focus on issues underpinning informed consent and different cultural and language needs.*

Domain: Nursing Practice and Decision Making

> 10. *All nurses must evaluate their care to improve clinical decision making, quality and outcomes, using a range of methods, amending the plan of care, where necessary, and communicating changes to others.*

Clinical decision making is a vital skill for student nurses to learn, as is finding ways to do it in a systematic way (Box 4.4) (Aston et al 2010).

To be able to make decisions that are safe and appropriate for the patient, yourself and others, you need to recognise different kinds of decisions you as a student may come across in a surgical placement. We now

---

Box 4.4 Domain: Nursing and Decision Making

Generic Competence

1. All nurses must use up-to-date knowledge and evidence to assess, plan, deliver and evaluate care, communicate findings, influence change and promote health and best practice. They must make person-centred, evidence-based judgements and decisions, in partnership with others involved in the care process, to ensure high-quality care. They must be able to recognise when the complexity of clinical decisions requires specialist knowledge and expertise, and consult or refer accordingly.

(NMC 2010:26)

consider some of these and determine what knowledge and skills you need to be able to act on these decision-making situations. These are areas you may need to revise prior to starting your clinical placement.

Note: we are talking generally here and this applies to any field of practice student who is undertaking a surgical placement.

Exposure to other fields of practice (or branches) is an absolutely essential part of your learning, and understanding the patient experience for example, from the point of view of someone with a mental health problem or who has learning difficulties undergoing surgery is relevant to all student nurses. In the main, this book focuses on adult surgery, as children have a very specific additional set of needs, although all the principles we discuss here are just as relevant to students experiencing a children's surgical placement.

Decision making in a surgical placement

On a daily basis, you will be working with either your mentor or other members of the team and learning from them how to care for patients having surgery for various reasons. Part of this care will involve using the nursing process stages or assessing, planning, implementing and evaluating care and, in many placements, using a nursing model as a framework for this. In some placements, you may encounter what is known as an integrated care pathway approach where all healthcare professionals caring for the patient have an opportunity to record their decisions regarding their input into patient care. It is important to note at this point that all qualified nurses are accountable for any decisions they make with regards to patient care. As a student, you are also responsible for your actions and must work towards being professionally accountable.

 Tip

Read the guidance on professional conduct for students (NMC 2009) again to ensure you fully understand these issues and discuss the meaning and implications for you as a student with your personal tutor.

Consider the following situations during the assessment stage of the nursing process when you might be required to make a decision and then consider what kinds of decision-making models these are based on (Box 4.5).

Activity

What kind of decision making is taking place in the following brief scenarios and how can you learn to prepare for such events or similar ones in your field of practice or generally?

1. A qualified nurse with 10 years' experience of working on a surgical ward has brought a patient back from theatre and has been taking his observations half hourly. These have been within normal parameters for a patient just returned from theatre. She has come to his bed to give him sips of water which he is now allowed, and sees that he is pale, rather restless and a bit breathless. She immediately tells the student nurse that the patient is bleeding somewhere. (There is nothing at this stage to indicate this directly as his signs and symptoms could be due to other things as well.)

Continued

Kind of decision making: intuition.

Up to this point, all she has done is look at the patient, drawn on her experience of caring for similar patients and decided that in her 'expert' view he is bleeding somewhere rather than anything else.

2. On that ward, there is a protocol to follow if a patient exhibits certain behaviours or signs such as those above, for all patients who have had major surgery, in the first 4 hours postoperatively.

The qualified nurse immediately puts this into action: take all observations, temperature, pulse and respirations plus blood pressure and, if showing significant signs of change from the previous pattern, inform the doctor immediately (for example if the blood pressure has dropped from 120/70 mmHg to 70/50 mmHg and there is a raised pulse of 130 beats per minute). Then the protocol requires that all wounds, drains, dressings are checked. At the same time, the patient should be asked if he is in pain.

Kind of decision making: information processing.

In undertaking all these activities, the nurse is gathering various cues and information regarding the physiological status of the patient as well as the physical and psychological status.

3. In observing his wound and dressing, the qualified nurse can see only a small amount of blood on the surface that would be expected on the dressing of someone who has had major surgery 3 hours previously. The patient, however, still has the same cues and she still believes he is showing signs of a serious bleed. At this stage, she uses her clinical judgement and decides to ask the student to help her turn the patient onto his side. Underneath the patient and soaking the sheet is evidence of a large loss of blood.

A normal response when asked to follow a protocol is to check everything on the list or pathway of decision making, as this is one which covers all patients as a benchmark for determining what is happening. It is information gathering. However, what the qualified nurse has done is use the cognitive continuum model where both types of decision making can work together in order to make the most effective and, in this case, urgent reassessment of the patient's situation. This allows the surgeon to make a clinical decision on whether to take the patient back to the operating theatre immediately in order to resolve the postoperative bleeding.

Box 4.5 Decision-making theories (based on Thompson & Dowding 2002)

Information-processing model

This framework, like others, has key steps to making decisions in practice. The first step is gathering preliminary clinical information about the patient, which can be considered as picking up cues (cue acquisition). This can be linked to the first stage of the nursing process, where you assess a patient's needs using a nursing model framework, e.g. the Roper, Logan and Tierney model (Holland et al 2008). Some of this information might be picked up before you even meet a patient and may come from a range of other places and people (see Ch. 5 on pre-admission assessment).

Box 4.5 Decision-making theories (based on Thompson & Dowding 2002)—cont'd

The second step is to develop some idea of what is wrong or what a patient's needs are from this information (e.g. health problems, signs and symptoms) and also to make a possible nursing diagnosis or hypothesis about what the problems might be.

The third step is to interpret all these cues and measure them against what you think is the problem; this is known as 'the reasoning process (interpretation)' (Thompson & Dowding, 2002:10).

The final step involves 'weighing up all the pros and cons of each possible explanation for your patient's signs and symptoms and other information gathered' (2002:10) and choosing an option that is based on the most evidence you have.

This kind of decision-making process may at first seem very structured for someone new to nursing, but as you gain more experience of similar situations and health problems, you will begin to link some cues to information in your memory bank of previous experiences, both in nursing and in your personal life.

The intuition model

Some of you will already have heard experienced qualified nurses say 'I just know there is something wrong' or 'I have a gut feeling about this situation'. They cannot, however, offer an explanation at the time of how they know, or the knowledge that goes with this knowing. Thompson and Dowding (2002:10) state that *'despite variations in the definition, there are commonalties in that intuition is perceived to be a process of reasoning that just happens; that cannot be examined and that is not rational'*. You may already have come across the idea of intuitive decision making in the work of Patricia Benner (1984), and some of you may have phrases from her work such as novice, advanced beginner and (developing) expert included in your assessment documents.

The cognitive continuum model

Making decisions in nursing practice is often a combination of the models above. A model that demonstrates how this can happen, is one where there is range of decision-making situations based on different types of evidence, in other words a continuum or range of decisions from intuition, where there is no immediate evidence seen other than the 'experience' of the nurse, to one where there is clearly a series of evidence cues enabling clear decisions to be made, possibly using some kind of 'decision-making tree' or pathway. In some surgical placements, you will come across processes called protocols which are, in basic terms, steps laid down which are to be followed when making a decision for a range of situations. These protocols are normally evidence based, and examples include clinical procedure steps for infection control practice or a directive for a major disaster. A study by Rycroft-Malone et al (2009) showed that qualified nurses used other kinds of information to help them make decisions even where protocol-based care was in place, and showed a range of decisions rather than following a standardised approach. When you are in your placement, there may be an opportunity to contribute to making decisions which will impact on patient care, but also learning to make decisions as part of your developing leadership and management role is essential for a qualified nurse.

Domain: Leadership, Management and Team Working

> 5. *All nurses must facilitate nursing students and others to develop their competence, using a range of professional and personal development skills.*

If you are a first year student, you might look at this competence and think 'I am never going to be able to do that until I'm in my third year'. You are correct in a way, as that is one of the competencies you will have to achieve by completion of your programme to be signed off in practice placement as being 'fit for practice' as a qualified nurse.

However, even as a first year student, there are skills that you can learn to work towards this, and learning something new and showing another student at the same stage as you how to do it is a good way of learning. This could be in the clinical skills laboratory first, then during the placement.

An excellent example, and one that students will definitely need to learn to undertake on a surgical placement, is that of taking a patient's blood pressure – both electronically and manually. Using both is an essential component of the Essential Skills Cluster: Organisational Aspects of Care (9), where it makes clear that before students can progress to the second part of their programme, they need to be able to accurately undertake and record a baseline assessment of blood pressure using manual and electronic devices (NMC 2010:113).

Use the following resource to remind you how to take a blood pressure reading and consider how you would then show and explain this to another student underpinned by an evidence base: http://www.bhsoc.org/how_to_measure_blood_pressure.stm (accessed December 2011). This facilitates the development of their competence in one thing while developing your competence in another. It is also helpful to prepare yourself by reading through notes you already have from lectures or from skills teaching sessions, so that you feel you know something before going to placement. (See also Ch. 14 in Brooker & Waugh 2007.)

Summary

We have seen that as well as preparing for what to expect from a surgical placement, it is also essential that you prepare yourself as a developing professional and student who has to be successful in achieving your assessment of practice and competencies for the NMC and eventually the register as a qualified nurse. This chapter has given you some examples of how to facilitate some of your learning in these areas and additional information is also found throughout the book to supplement and add to the guidance in this section.

References

Arkell, S., Bayliss Pratt, L., 2007. How nursing students can make the most out of their placements. Online. Available at: http://www.nursingtimes.net/nursing-practice-clinical-research/how-nursing-students-can-make-the-most-of-placements/199226.article (accessed September 2011).

Aston, L., Wakefield, J., McGowan, R., 2010. The student nurse guide to decision making in practice. Open University Press, Maidenhead.

Benner, P., 1984. From novice to expert. Addison–Wesley, California.

Brooker, C., Waugh, A., 2007. Foundations of nursing practice: fundamentals of holistic care. Mosby, Edinburgh.

Buchan, J., O'May, F., Little, L., 2008. Review of models of employment for nursing roles which bridge practice and education. A report for NHS Education for Scotland, Queen Margaret University, Edinburgh.

Carlisle, C., Calman, L., Ibbotson, T., 2009. Practice-based learning: the role of practice education facilitators in supporting mentors. Nurse Education Today 29 (7), 715–721.

Fowler, J., 1998. The handbook of clinical supervision: your questions answered. Quay Books, Salisbury.

Holland, K., 2010. Utilising research and evidence based practice in assignment work. In: Holland, K., Rees, C. (Eds.), Nursing: evidence-based practice skills. Oxford University Press, Oxford.

Holland, K., Rees, C., 2010. Nursing: evidence-based practice skills. Oxford University Press, Oxford.

Holland, K., Jenkins, J., Solomon, J., Whittam, S., 2008. Applying the Roper, Logan and Tierney model in practice. Churchill Livingstone, Edinburgh.

Levett-Jones, T., Bourgeois, S., 2009. The clinical placement. Baillière Tindall, Edinburgh.

Nursing and Midwifery Council, 2004. Standards for proficiency for pre-registration nursing education. NMC, London.

Nursing and Midwifery Council, 2007. Ensuring continuity of practice assessment through the ongoing achievement record. NMC, London.

Nursing and Midwifery Council, 2008. The code: standards of conduct, performance and ethics for nurses and midwives. NMC, London.

Nursing and Midwifery Council, 2009. Guidance on professional conduct for nursing and midwifery students. NMC, London.

Nursing and Midwifery Council, 2010a. Standards for pre-registration nursing education. NMC, London.

Nursing and Midwifery Council, 2010b. Good health and good character: guidance for approved educational institutions. NMC, London.

Por, J., Barriball, L., 2008. The personal tutor's role in pre-registration nursing education. British Journal of Nursing 13 (2), 99–103.

Pudner, R. (Ed.), 2010. Nursing the surgical patient, 3rd ed. Baillière Tindall, Edinburgh.

Roberts, D., 2010. How you will learn in practice. In: Hart, S. (Ed.), Nursing: study and placement learning skills. Oxford University Press, Oxford.

Rycroft-Malone, J., Fontenla, M., Seers, K., Bick, D., 2009. Protocol-based care: the standardisation of decision making? J. Clin. Nurs. 18, 1490–1500.

Thompson, C., Dowding, D., 2002. Decision making and judgement in nursing – an introduction. In: Thompson, C., Dowding, D. (Eds.), Clinical decision making and judgement in nursing. Churchill Livingstone, Edinburgh.

Timmins, F., 2008. Making sense of portfolios – a guide for nursing students. Open University Press, Maidenhead.

Further reading

Donaldson, J., Ness, V., 2009. Maintaining a safe environment. In: Docherty, C., McCallum, J. (Eds.), Foundation clinical nursing skills. Oxford University Press, Oxford.

Gilmour, D., 2010. Perioperative care. In: Pudner, R. (Ed.), Nursing the surgical patient, 3rd ed. Baillière Tindall, Edinburgh.

Waugh, A., Grant, A., 2010. Ross and Wilson anatomy and physiology: colouring and workbook, 3rd ed. Churchill Livingstone, Edinburgh.

Websites

There are a number of publications for student nurses at the RCN website which are helpful to read prior to undertaking any clinical placement experience. Access this link for these publications: http://www.rcn.org.uk/development/publications/publicationsA-Z?78808_result_page=H#H (accessed December 2011).

1. *Helping Students Get the Best from their Practice Placements* (RCN 2002). Please keep in mind when reading this that the NMC has amended their standards for pre-registration nursing education (NMC 2010a).

2. *An Ageing Population: Education and Practice Preparation for Nursing Students Learning to Work with Older People* (RCN 2008). A resource pack for nursing students. A very useful publication based on a research project which will help students understand the specific needs of older people in any healthcare setting.

3. *Benchmarks for Children's Orthopaedic Nursing Care* (RCN 2007). An excellent publication relating to children's nursing care in an orthopaedic context which also has sections relating to surgical nursing and pre- and postoperative care.

4. *Dignity in Health Care for People with Learning Disabilities (RCN 2010)*. Another excellent publication offering examples of best practice in caring for people with learning disabilities in various healthcare settings, including being in hospital.

5. *Dyslexia, Dyspraxia and Dyscalculia: a Toolkit for Nursing Staff (RCN 2010)*. This is an RCN publication that has been developed for students as well as qualified nurses and others and, in particular, a supportive one which is reassuring for any student with any of these three learning difficulties to negotiate assistance before and during placement.

Section 2. Placement learning opportunities

In this section, we take you on a journey through each possible stage of a patient's experience of undergoing a surgical procedure. It is anticipated that you will meet with your mentor to discuss the learning opportunities available in the placement. It may be that a model of a 'hub and spoke'/insight visit placement exists or maybe you have one main base placement from which to experience a range of linked experiences for various lengths of time.

This could be a short 6-week placement or as long as 18 weeks over a year of learning. Following the introduction of the new Nursing and Midwifery Council standards, you may experience 'placement learning pathways' (see Chs 3 and 4), which will be a combined placement following a possible journey that a patient might experience (see Section 3). In addition, there may be opportunities to experience other learning opportunities such as seeing what a pharmacist does and how a dietician helps people recover from surgery.

Whatever length of time your placement is, the chapters in this section help you to plan your placement learning opportunities and give those of you who are unable to follow a patient through their whole experience an insight into aspects of that journey in order to understand it better.

In this section, the placement learning pathway follows a typical surgical patient's journey. Linked to each stage are areas where you may undertake either a full placement experience or insight/spoke placements.

5 Pre-admission assessment of the patient and discharge planning

CHAPTER AIMS

- To explore the underpinning philosophy of pre-admission assessment
- To explore the actual experience of a pre-admission assessment
- To increase awareness of the role that pre-admission assessment plays in patient safety and comfort when admitted to hospital for surgery
- To provide an evidence-based foundation for pre-admission assessment

Introduction

Traditionally and historically, many professionals within the hospital environment have been involved in the assessment of patients going for surgery. These include medical staff, nurses, pharmacists and physiotherapists. Individually, each professional would 'assess' the patient from their individual professional perspective (Bassett 2005). As a result, the patient would have to repeat similar information to a number of professionals. The impact of this was that vital information was often lost. Recognition of this and the need to continually improve and streamline patient services has become the result. A major development that we have seen over the last 7–10 years has been in the area of multi-professional assessment services. In particular the learning gained from the early work of day surgery units and the guidelines and practices these adapted to patient selection.

Almost 40 years ago, Crosby et al (1972) researched the benefits of pre-admission assessment on surgical patients and recommended that such assessments should take place. Undoubtedly, for many years, organisations interpreted the aims of pre-admission assessment in different ways and gave such services varying amounts of support (Bassett 2005). It only became apparent how important such a service could be with the reduction in working hours of junior doctors (Department of Health (DH) 1997) as this change resulted in a lack of time to 'clerk' patients traditionally. This presented the idea that professionals other than doctors should become involved in the process. Nevertheless, owing to a lack of leadership from key stakeholders anxious to ensure that their professional identity was maintained and anxious not to make recommendations for other professional groups, little was written on the subject until the NHS Modernisation Agency published national guidelines in 2003.

Equally, as the focus of healthcare delivery has shifted from inpatient to ambulatory care and the need to treat greater numbers of patients, healthcare organisations have had to review/develop assessment services which are able to meet these demands.

The recognition of the contribution this model of assessment can offer to organisations and patients has clearly been articulated by the Scottish Executive (2005) in the strategy document *Building a Health Service Fit for the Future*. A key to successful assessment in a modernising NHS is that:

> at all times it must be evident to the patient that despite the large number of individuals involved, they are all working together and are in possession of all relevant information. Their individual roles, training and responsibilities should be clear to patients.
>
> (Scottish Executive 2005:14)

Key drivers for pre-admission assessment

Pre-admission assessment clinics are now commonplace for surgical specialties. Pre-admission assessment is the process of assessing patients prior to surgery. The key purpose of this assessment is to reduce perioperative morbidity and mortality by identifying patients who may require further assessment, investigation or treatment of co-morbidity prior to surgery (Janke et al 2002).

Activity

Provide your own definition of pre-admission assessment.

Consider and write down why pre-admission assessment is necessary for patients prior to coming into hospital.

This definition of pre-operative assessment by NHS Scotland (2008:4) may help you to consider this activity:

> Pre-operative assessment establishes that the patient is fully informed and wishes to undergo the procedure. It ensures that the patient is as fit as possible for the surgery and anaesthetic. It minimises the risk of late cancellations by ensuring that all essential resources and discharge requirements are identified and coordinated.

The main driving force behind this change has been the acknowledgement that patient-centred assessment services have become a key means of how the NHS can deliver on national targets (DoH 2001). Nationally, the main drivers for this change were the Labour Government NHS modernisation agenda (pre-2009) and the National Institute for Health and Clinical Excellence (NICE) guidelines for preoperative testing (2003), the aims being to reduce last minute cancellations and to be able to facilitate day of surgery admissions.

Activity

Follow this link to obtain evidence of the NHS Modernisation Agency (2002) *National Good Practice Guidance on Pre-operative Assessment for Day Surgery*:

http://www.generalsurgerybirmingham .co.uk/documents/gen-vasc-guidelines/Microsoft%20Word%20-%20guidance%20copeland%2019.pdf (accessed May 2011).

and the (2003) *National Good Practice Guidance on Pre-operative Assessment for In-patient Surgery*:

http://uat.qihub.scot.nhs.uk/quality-healthcare-resources/continuous-improvement-in-healthcare/

improvement-tools/search-results/
improvement-tool.aspx?id=71
(Accessed May 2012).

Read the documents and write out three learning goals that you can achieve if you are in a pre-admission clinic for your clinical placement, e.g. you might consider the informed consent needs of patients from different cultures and learn about the specific cultural needs of one of these groups that will help you plan their care.

These documents are essential reading for this Section of the book and will also help you in Sections 3 and 4.

Historically, within surgery, patients were not always adequately prepared for general anaesthetic due to either inadequate preoperative testing or patients being classified as unfit for surgery. In some cases, this led to operations being cancelled and operating department ineffectiveness. Pre-assessment was performed 1–2 weeks prior to admission resulting in such cancellations because some identified health problems could not always be resolved in the time before surgery and hospital admission.

Following the introduction of the two national good practice guidance documents, single pre-admission assessment clinics were introduced and followed a radically revised care pathway. When a decision for elective surgery is made, within the outpatient department, the patient is immediately taken for anaesthetic assessment. All the necessary preoperative investigations are completed in accordance with the NICE guidelines for preoperative testing (NICE 2003). Objectives of preoperative assessment (NHS Modernisation Agency 2003) prior to inpatient surgery are listed in Box 5.1 and this offers an excellent overview for you to help plan learning outcomes.

Who conducts the pre-admission assessment?

At present it is a registered nurse who completes the nursing assessment and a doctor who completes the medical assessment. As changes are made to the education and training of doctors and with the reduction in working hours of junior doctors (Oakley & Bratchell 2010), nurses are taking on more of the junior doctors' role and, certainly in the UK, there are nurse specialists in this field (DH 2006).

In the case of day surgery/ambulatory surgery, trained nurses undertake the complete assessment. Doctors will see the patient on the day of surgery for medical checks and to obtain consent (see Ch. 6 for issues around informed consent).

The good practice guidelines recommended that preoperative assessment for either day surgery or inpatient surgery should be 'performed by a trained and competent preoperative assessor' (NHS Modernisation Agency 2003:6). Each NHS trust or independent hospital will have its own practice guidelines and policies with regards to this, and if you are in a pre-admission placement, it would be good practice to read this and be familiar with the content as patients may ask you: 'Who is going to see me today? Is it the doctor?' It requires a multidisciplinary team approach to ensure seamless care for patients.

When a problem is identified, such as a patient having a cold or a chest infection, which may result in a patient's surgery being cancelled or where further advice is required, an anaesthetist is contacted so that decisions can be made regarding the management of the patient either pre- or postoperatively. The anaesthetist may have dedicated pre-admission sessions and be available most days for either patient or notes review. The anaesthetist also sees the patient on the morning of surgery if the patient is for day surgery or ambulatory care

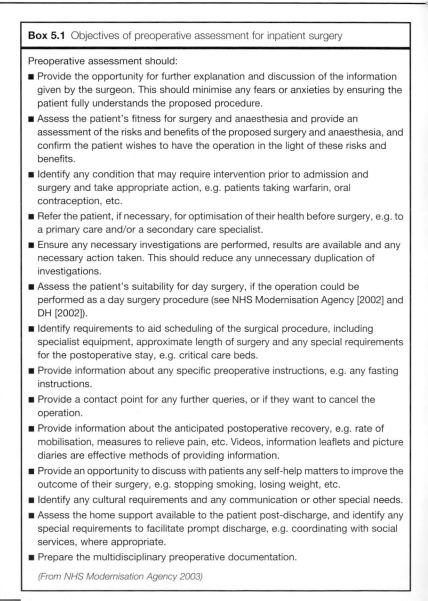

Box 5.1 Objectives of preoperative assessment for inpatient surgery

Preoperative assessment should:

- Provide the opportunity for further explanation and discussion of the information given by the surgeon. This should minimise any fears or anxieties by ensuring the patient fully understands the proposed procedure.
- Assess the patient's fitness for surgery and anaesthesia and provide an assessment of the risks and benefits of the proposed surgery and anaesthesia, and confirm the patient wishes to have the operation in the light of these risks and benefits.
- Identify any condition that may require intervention prior to admission and surgery and take appropriate action, e.g. patients taking warfarin, oral contraception, etc.
- Refer the patient, if necessary, for optimisation of their health before surgery, e.g. to a primary care and/or a secondary care specialist.
- Ensure any necessary investigations are performed, results are available and any necessary action taken. This should reduce any unnecessary duplication of investigations.
- Assess the patient's suitability for day surgery, if the operation could be performed as a day surgery procedure (see NHS Modernisation Agency [2002] and DH [2002]).
- Identify requirements to aid scheduling of the surgical procedure, including specialist equipment, approximate length of surgery and any special requirements for the postoperative stay, e.g. critical care beds.
- Provide information about any specific preoperative instructions, e.g. any fasting instructions.
- Provide a contact point for any further queries, or if they want to cancel the operation.
- Provide information about the anticipated postoperative recovery, e.g. rate of mobilisation, measures to relieve pain, etc. Videos, information leaflets and picture diaries are effective methods of providing information.
- Provide an opportunity to discuss with patients any self-help matters to improve the outcome of their surgery, e.g. stopping smoking, losing weight, etc.
- Identify any cultural requirements and any communication or other special needs.
- Assess the home support available to the patient post-discharge, and identify any special requirements to facilitate prompt discharge, e.g. coordinating with social services, where appropriate.
- Prepare the multidisciplinary preoperative documentation.

(From NHS Modernisation Agency 2003)

surgery. For patients having inpatient surgery or planned surgery, they may see the patient the day before as the majority are admitted at least the day before surgery is to take place (see Ch. 6). The good practice guide also gives an overview of the guidelines used for selecting patients for day surgery, including when day surgery would not be considered, e.g. pain cannot be controlled with oral analgesia and specific physiological contraindications such as poorly controlled asthma or having had a heart attack in the last 6 months.

◎ Activity

Identify three other situations where a patient might not be considered suitable for day surgery.

Identify what kind of investigations might be considered for patients during the pre-admission assessment.

Identify at least two investigations where you could visit, with a patient's permission, to understand what these involve.

Depending on the type of surgery a patient is having, other members of the multidisciplinary team may also be involved in the pre-admission assessment process. For example, a physiotherapist might assess a patient's needs and give advice regarding exercise regimes and mobilising in the postoperative period (see section on nursing assessment on admission to hospital in Ch. 6).

Referral to an occupational therapist may be required, who assesses the patient's requirements for discharge home from hospital: for example they may be required not to climb stairs or require raised toilet seats. Patients who are having joint replacements are asked to complete a form, which records the height of chairs, bed and so forth so that any identified requirements

are dealt with prior to the patient's discharge home (see Royal National Orthopaedic Hospital leaflet on total hip replacement: http://www.rnoh.nhs.uk/sites/default/files/downloads/10-86_rnoh_pg_thr_web_0.pdf (accessed May 2011)).

A pharmacist may see a patient to address any problems with medications while they are in hospital. For example, a patient may be an insulin-dependent diabetic or taking steroids, both of which will be affected by surgery. For patients coming to hospital for day surgery/ambulatory surgery, the nurse will complete a pharmacy pre-assessment sheet and send it for the attention of the pharmacist.

The consultant surgeon, surgical registrar or surgical care practitioner will ideally be available for the pre-assessment visit to explain the procedure to the patient and get the consent form signed. They would also be able to ensure that any questions that accompanying relatives have can be answered. A useful document to read in relation to patients with learning difficulties who may require surgery is that written specifically for nurses by the Royal College of Nursing (RCN 2006).

◎ Activity

Consider the process of assessment that patients in your placement area have undergone in the pre-admission clinic and identify the main health problems that may have been identified.

Re-visit who is involved in the pre-admission assessment and what their role is with regards to patient care.

Consider how information gathered is communicated to other professionals involved with the patient.

Discuss these issues with your mentor as part of your planned learning plan.

Key components of good pre-admission assessment

The major goal of pre-assessment services is to assess the holistic needs of patients and determine their suitability for surgery (Johansson et al 2010). The information obtained enables the team to engage with careful patient selection and plan individual care accordingly.

 Activity

> Read the articles by Beck (2007) and Gilmartin (2004) (see References), related to pre-admission nursing assessments, prior to your surgical placement as background to understanding the nurse's role in this critical area of patient care in the pre-operative period.

The Scottish Executive (2005) noted that failure to assess patients adequately can be responsible for high operating theatre cancellation rates, or unacceptable risks to patients. It further advises that studies in Australia have shown that inadequate assessment is frequently implicated in deaths attributable to anaesthesia (Mackay 2004).

Traditionally, pre-admission assessment services were delivered within the hospital environment. With the modernisation of services along with advances in technology, opportunities exist for pre-admission services to be delivered in more innovative ways (NHS Modernisation Agency 2003:10). Some innovative ways in which pre-admission services are being delivered are the following:

- In patients' homes.
- Within primary care.
- At one-stop clinics.
- Via a telephone service.
- Via digital television (telemedicine).
- Postal questionnaires.

Many advocates of pre-admission assessment services believe there is a place for using information technology in assessment (Macduff et al 2001). In some facilities, information is stored directly on a database and shared between the relevant professionals. In others, patients hold their own records and take them to where they are needed. In both cases, assessment is a good example of the opportunities for sharing information among professionals, and this will only improve with the advent of the electronic patient record (Scottish Executive 2005).

Whatever the method of delivering pre-admission assessment services, it must always be appropriate to the patient and the type of surgery they will undergo.

 Activity

> Consider what aspects of pre-admission assessment are routinely undertaken in preparing patients for surgery/investigation in your clinical placement.
>
> Discuss this with your mentor and consider how you can gain an insight into how a pre-admission clinic or assessment works.

No matter where pre-admission assessment services are delivered, the NHS Modernisation Agency (2003:5) detail key objectives for pre-assessment services as follows:

Confirmation the patient wishes to have the recommended procedure/investigation.

- *Assess the patient's suitability to be treated as either an inpatient, day case patient or ambulatory care patient.*
- *Assess the patient's fitness for the surgery/investigation.*
- *Ensure the patient fully comprehends what the procedure/investigation will entail and provide additional oral and written information.*

- *Take the opportunity to minimise any anxiety or fears the patient may have.*
- *Identify any special requirements the patient may have.*
- *Provide the opportunity for discussion in relation to self-help matters to improve the outcomes (e.g. smoking cessation, losing weight).*
- *Identify any cultural requirements.*
- *Identify problems in advance so that they can be addressed.*
- *Allow the patient to make suitable arrangements for work, childcare, etc.*
- *Ensure the patient will be able to go home safely.*
- *Reduce preventable cancellations on the day of surgery.*
- *Provide a smooth admission process to avoid delays on the day of surgery.*
- *Predict and explain risks to patients.*
- *Assess the home support available to the patient and identify any special requirements to facilitate prompt discharge.*

To achieve the above objectives, the following assessments will be required.

The nursing pre-admission assessment process

A careful and detailed history and clinical examination are essential to ensure that important information is not omitted which could have an impact on the pre- and postoperative care of a patient. The aim of the history taking is to obtain and document a complete picture of a patient's present health problems alongside their past medical history, family history and social circumstances. All pre-admission assessment services gather this information via a standard document based upon the NICE (2003) guidelines for preoperative testing: http://www.nice.org.uk/nicemedia/live/10920/29090/29090.pdf (accessed December 2011).

Activity

Before continuing with this chapter, read the NMC (2010) Standard related to the requirements of the Essential Skills cluster of care, compassion and communication (Box 5.2). Consider how you will achieve these essential skills by setting yourself objectives while learning about pre-admission assessment. Discuss with your mentor how she/he will assess your skills and competencies to meet both outcomes. An example of what is required can be seen in Box 5.3 (See NMC Standard 6).

Box 5.2 Essential Skills Cluster: Care, Compassion and Communication

Standard 6

People can trust the newly registered graduate nurse to engage therapeutically and actively listen to their needs and concerns, responding using skills that are helpful, providing information that is clear, accurate, meaningful and free from jargon. (NMC, 2010)

The newly qualified graduate nurse should demonstrate the skills and behaviours shown in Box 5.3: they should be used to develop learning outcomes for each progression point and for outcomes to be achieved before entering the register.

Communication with the patient

We can see from the Essential Skills Cluster and NMC (2010) Standard the importance of being able to communicate effectively with patients.

Box 5.3 Requirements to achieve NMC Competencies at the three Progression Points to becoming a nurse

First progression point	Second progression point	Transfer to the register
1. Communicates effectively both orally and in writing, so that the meaning is always clear	6. Uses strategies to enhance communication and remove barriers to effective communication, minimising risk to people from lack of or poor communication	7. Consistently shows ability to communicate safely and effectively with people, providing guidance for others
2. Records information accurately and clearly on the basis of observation and communication		8. Communicates effectively and sensitively in different settings, using a range of methods and skills
3. Always seeks to confirm understanding		9. Provides accurate and comprehensive written and verbal reports based on best available evidence
4. Responds in a way that confirms what a person is communicating		10. Acts autonomously to reduce and challenge barriers to effective communication and understanding
5. Effectively communicates people's stated needs and wishes to other professionals		11. Is proactive and creative in enhancing communication and understanding
		12. Uses the skills of active listening, questioning, paraphrasing and reflection to support a therapeutic intervention
		13. Uses appropriate and relevant communication skills to deal with difficult and challenging circumstances, for example responding to emergencies, unexpected occurrences, saying 'no', dealing with complaints, de-escalating agression, conveying 'unwelcome news'

When conducting any assessment with a patient for the first time, it is important always to introduce yourself. It is also important to ask the patient how they would like you to address them (e.g. by their first name or as Mr Smith). Even this may not be appropriate for some cultures (see Holland & Hogg (2010) for cultural names).

Throughout the assessment, it is important to maintain eye contact at all times with the patient, to speak slowly and clearly when asking questions and to allow the patient time to answer questions. For patients whose first language is not English, it is important to ensure that either a family member who does speak English is present or to ensure that an interpreter is available. For patients with hearing or language impairment, many hospital services can provide 'sign language' experts to assist. (See http://www.nmhdu.org.uk/our-work/ mhep/accessible-mental-health-services/ (accessed December 2011) for information and other links.)

Prior to carrying out the assessment, it is important to ensure that any previous medical records and X-rays are available for you to review as well as being available to the surgeon/anesthetist if required.

Personal details

To set the patient at ease, it is helpful to start with asking simple questions such as to confirm their full name, their date of birth, address, marital status, occupation, contact details for next of kin, religion/spiritual beliefs and ethnic background. If the patient has medical notes then the details provided by the patient should be checked with those held on the medical records.

Existing medical conditions

During pre-admission assessment (which is unlike a nursing assessment normally undertaken on admission to a ward, for example), it is very important to systematically go through each of the body's systems and elicit and document if the patient has any conditions which are being treated. The pre-admission checklists used in pre-admission assessment services will help guide you through this. The most common areas to explore are in relation to the following:

- Cardiac system: do they have angina, hypertension, ischaemic heart disease? Have they ever had coronary artery bypass surgery?
- Respiratory system: respiratory tract infections, chronic obstructive pulmonary disease, asthma, bronchitis.
- Central nervous system: do they have epilepsy? Have they ever had a stroke or transient ischaemic attack (TIA), Parkinson's disease, dementia? Determine if there are any addictions such as alcohol dependence or recreational drug use.
- Renal system: do they have frequent urinary tract infections? Have they ever had renal failure? Do they have diabetes?
- Hepatobiliary system: have they ever had hepatitis, cirrhosis of the liver?
- Gastrointestinal system: Have they ever had oesophageal reflux, anorexia, nausea?
- Reproductive system: if female and of childbearing years, is their menstrual cycle regular?
- Haematological system: do they have anaemia, haemophilia? Do they take anticoagulation or antiplatelet medications.
- Musculoskeletal system: do they have arthritis and/or restricted neck or joint movement.

✓ Tip

To learn more about preoperative tests and investigations, access the following document from NICE: http://www.nice.org.uk/nicemedia/ live/10920/29090/29090.pdf (accessed December 2011).

In addition to the above, it is important to ask the patient if they have had contact with anyone or have themselves had methicillin-resistant *Staphylococcus aureus* (MRSA) recently and been in hospital over the last 3 months. If they answer yes to any of these questions, they may require an MRSA screen. This is particularly necessary for any patient, for example, who is to have a prosthesis inserted, due to the potential risk of postoperative infection.

Medications

It is important to document all medications that the patient is currently on, including medications which have been prescribed. Pay particular attention to the route of administration, dosage and how frequently the medication is taken. It is also important to ask the patient specifically if they are taking any herbal medicines as many herbal medicines can interact with prescribed medications and anaesthetic medications. You should document the name and also how often the patient takes these.

A further area to elicit information on is around the use of recreational drugs. You must document the name, how much they take and the frequency with which they use any recreational drugs. Many recreational drugs like herbal medications can have an adverse reaction with anaesthetic drugs. It is crucial to draw any usage of herbal medications and recreational drugs to the attention of the anaesthetists.

Allergies

Ask about and document any allergies the patient has. It is important to find out not only if they have allergies to any medications but also to any foods, for example peanuts, bananas or kiwi fruits, as these food allergies can be a result of having an undiagnosed allergy to latex rubber. Ask the patient what happens when their allergy is triggered, for example sneezing, vomiting, skin rash (further detailed information is given in Ch. 6). All allergies must be communicated to the anaesthetist directly.

Investigations

There are a number of routine investigations that are carried out on all patients. These usually begin with recording a patient's baseline temperature, pulse and respirations (TPR) and blood pressure (BP). This provides a baseline of the patient's normal parameters.

Recording height and weight then allows the body mass index (BMI) to be calculated. The BMI is a statistical measure that compares a person's weight and height. It is also used to estimate a healthy body weight based on a person's height and this has already been worked out for you on a recognised BMI chart. This is a widely used diagnostic tool and can identify if someone is underweight, overweight or obese. For example, in the UK, a patient with a BMI over 35 is not suitable for day surgery. (See http://www.nhs.uk/Tools/Pages/Healthyweightcalculator.aspx for tools to calculate BMI and links to related health problems. It is also linked to a range of health and wellbeing and weight management resources.)

> **◈ Activity**
>
> Using the *British National Formulary* (BNF), identify three common herbal medications and how they could interact with other traditional medications prescribed.

> **◈ Activity**
>
> Using the BMI chart, practice the clinical skill of calculating patients' BMI and recording this on your local care planning documentation. If unsure

if you have calculated correctly, check with your mentor. Knowing a patient's normal height and weight measurement on admission to hospital is essential if you are to calculate the patient's BMI. This would not of course be possible in emergency admission to hospital.

Routine urinalysis is carried out primarily to ensure that the patient has no infection or undiagnosised diabetes mellitus. It is particularly important for patients going for joint replacement surgery or having insertion of metal work to be free from infection, as any infection can get into the prosthesis and cause it to fail.

A pregnancy test should be carried out on all female patients of childbearing age who continue to menstruate. It is highly dangerous to a foetus to administer a general anaesthetic.

⊗ Activity

If you are in a pre-admission clinic placement, under the supervision of your mentor, conduct a pre admission assessment of one patient. After completing this, make a list of what you felt you did well and areas you feel you require further practice in. Compare your own assessment with the assessment your mentor made. What did you find was different and what knowledge and skills do you need to develop?

If you are not allocated to a pre-admission clinic, ensure that you devise a **SMART** (**S**pecific, **M**easurable, **A**chievable, **R**ealistic and **T**imely) objective in relation to negotiating an insight learning day or hub and spoke placement.

Additional investigations such as an electrocardiogram (ECG), blood tests and X-rays may be undertaken depending on the patient's medical history. For example, an ECG may be required if the patient has a heart condition. Many pre-admission assessment services have algorithms to help make a decision as to whether a patient requires an ECG.

Anaesthetic history

It is extremely useful to know if a patient has had an anaesthetic in the past and whether they had any problems. If a patient has had a previous anaesthetic and tells you they had a problem with it, it is important to document the exact nature of the problem. The most common problem is severe nausea and vomiting after the anaesthetic. It is important to record any problem voiced by the patient and draw this to the attention of the anaesthetist. Knowing if a patient has had a previous anaesthetic problem allows for planning better postoperative care. There are also conditions which run in families that are extremely dangerous if not managed properly that may manifest when a patient is anaesthetised (e.g. malignant hyperpyrexia).

All of the above mainly relate to the physical fitness of a patient. All patients undergoing a surgical intervention are also assessed in relation to their American Society of Anesthesiologists (ASA) physical status. ASA physical status is a physical fitness tool developed by the ASA and used routinely around the world. It is divided into six levels:

- *ASA 1: a normal healthy patient.*
- *ASA 2: a patient with mild systemic disease – an example of this is a patient that has diabetes mellitus that is controlled by diet only.*
- *ASA 3: a patient with severe systemic disease – an example of this is a patient with diabetes mellitus who requires insulin but whose blood glucose level is well controlled.*

- *ASA 4: a patient with severe systemic disease that is a constant threat to life – an example of this is a patient with diabetes mellitus who requires insulin but whose blood glucose level is not well controlled and who has frequent episodes of hypoglycaemia which requires medical attention.*
- *ASA 5: a moribund patient who is not expected to survive without the operation.*
- *ASA 6: a declared brain-dead patient whose organs are being removed for donor purposes.*

The ASA status of a patient determines whether they will be treated as an inpatient, day case patient or ambulatory patient. Routinely, patients who have an ASA of 1 or 2 can be treated as a day case and patients with an ASA 3 can be treated on an ambulatory basis. Patients who score above ASA 3 are always treated as inpatients as there is an increased risk of requiring either intensive or high-dependency care following surgery.

Anaesthetists have the ultimate authority on a patient's suitability for anaesthesia and there are processes in place to allow nursing staff to communicate findings to anaesthetic staff and to seek guidance from them.

Surgical factors

Any surgical operation causes physiological stress to a patient. The physiological stress becomes greater the more invasive a procedure is. There is no universally agreed and validated scoring system for classifying the 'stress' of a procedure. NICE (2003), however, has developed a simple grading scale:

- *Grade 1 (minor): examples include the removal of a simple skin lesion or drainage of a breast abscess.*
- *Grade 2 (intermediate): examples include removal of varicose leg veins, repair of an inguinal hernia.*
- *Grade 3 (major): examples include total abdominal hysterectomy, thyroidectomy.*

- *Grade 4 (major +): examples include neurosurgery, cardiac surgery, total joint replacement.*

Considerations should be given to the following key factors as part of the assessment process:

- Will the surgery involve significant blood loss or fluid shifts?
- Is the surgery associated with significant nausea and vomiting?
- Is the surgery associated with pain not treatable with simple analgesia?
- Is the surgery associated with prolonged immobilisation?

The above considerations determine whether a patient is admitted as a day case, ambulatory care or as an inpatient.

Social history

When conducting the social history, it is important to be aware that many patients take on a large part of their postoperative care themselves. It is important to find out about patients' social support networks. For example, do they live with someone or do they live alone? Are friends or family available and willing to help support them following discharge from hospital?

The type of housing is also a factor for consideration. For example, does the patient live in a high-rise block of flats where the lift is regularly out of order? For a patient having surgery to their leg, this may make it impossible for them to go home until fully mobile. Another factor to consider is how accessible their toilet is – is it up a flight of stairs? If having surgery that will limit their mobility, this could pose problems on discharge.

It is crucial to ascertain if there is a particular time of year that a patient is not available for admission for surgery. For example, they may be going away on holiday.

Also give consideration to the distance a patient must travel between the facility and home. Whether or not it is appropriate to allow a patient to travel home will also depend on the procedure and anaesthetic involved.

As identified earlier, some patients take on a large part of their postoperative care themselves; therefore it is important to consider the accessibility/availability of a telephone. This is crucial as many studies have found that, following discharge, patients still require advice, support and information in order for them to self-care.

Activity

Obtain a copy of one or both of the articles by Caroll and Dowling (2007) and Goodman (2010) (see References). Read and consider the importance of planning for discharge and who needs to be involved in this process. (See Ch. 10 for further information on discharge planning.)

Psychological assessment

A key aim of conducting a psychological assessment is to determine the level of knowledge and understanding patients have of the procedure they are about to have and the potential effects on their life. It is crucial to provide patients with accurate information so that they have realistic expectations about the surgery. For example, the removal of varicose leg veins does not mean that a patient will never have these again, but the patient may have been led to believe that the surgery will solve their problem indefinitely.

It is also important to assess any learning needs patients have and how these can be addressed prior to admission. Also determine which is the best medium to provide patients with further education, for example videos, pictures, leaflets, audio tapes.

All patients going for surgery are naturally anxious and worried. It is important to find out what worries they have and how we can assist to reduce these.

Activity

Two articles you will find helpful in understanding more about preoperative anxiety are Pritchard (2009) and Grieve (2002) (see References and also Further Reading). Discuss with your mentor the value of implementing care based on evidence of good practice in anxiety management.

Patient information

During pre-assessment, patients are given information to help them prepare for their admission to hospital. This information includes the following:
- What to bring into hospital including all medications in original packaging.
- What medications to take on the day of surgery and what medications to omit.
- Fasting instructions.
- Information for relatives.
- What to expect on the day of surgery.
- Postoperative care and instructions regarding time off work, mobility, etc.
- Information leaflets specific to the surgery they will have.
- Health promotion, e.g. weight reduction, stopping smoking.
- Ward contact details.

Evidence shows that if patients have a clear understanding of postoperative expectations, they recover more quickly and get home more quickly.

Activity

Read the articles by Johansson et al (2010) and Smith and Callery (2005) and consider the issues regarding patient information needs.

You may have an individual project to undertake for an assessment during your placement; one project could be to design an evidence-based preoperative admission leaflet for a patient who could be a child, an older person or someone with learning difficulties.

When you are observing your mentor undertaking a preoperative assessment or you are being observed, work out what you wish to learn from the experience. Preparation prior to placement is very helpful in enabling you to engage with patient care in any placement (see Chs 1–4).

Discharge planning

Discharge from hospital is a key element of a patient's stay, therefore planning for discharge must start before admission (Shepperd et al 2010). Much of the information required for efficient discharge planning will have been gathered during the social assessment of the patient. However, dependent on the type of surgery, the involvement of an occupational therapist and possibly social work referral may be required to establish, for example, the following:

- Does the patient's home need to be assessed?
- Will they need a raised toilet seat or hand rails?
- Will they require increased services such as meals on wheels, home help?
- How will they get home from hospital? If there is no friend or family member available, transport arrangements may be required.

(See Ch. 10 and the section on social history, above, for examples of articles that will help you understand the importance of discharge planning.)

> ✅ **Tip**
>
> Most hospitals have a discharge management team. Seek out further information on team members and how they support safe and timely hospital discharge for patients. Engage with team members as part of an insight learning day and make notes on their role.

Benefits of pre-admission assessment

Much of the literature demonstrates that pre-admission assessment services are beneficial in reducing hospital-led cancellations, patient-led cancellations and patients not attending (DH 2001). Some of the key benefits for both the patient and the service are:

Patient
- Ensures the patient is fit for surgery.
- Allows the patient to ask questions.
- Provides the patient with valuable information.
- Decreases fasting times.
- In paediatrics, some areas have pre-assessment parties which is beneficial both to the child and parents.

Service
- Prevents cancellation on the day of surgery.
- Allows better utilisation of beds.
- Reduces 'did not attend' (DNA) rate.
- Opportunity to give patients necessary information.
- Allows professionals to manage risk.
- Increases patient safety.
- Promotes multidisciplinary working.

When a pre-assessment is complete and the receiving ward is in receipt of this, it is then the responsibility of the ward staff to check the pre-assessment prior to a patient's admission, as very valuable information is contained in the document.

If a patient is pre-assessed for surgery and then has to wait up to 3–6 months for that surgery, it is necessary for the patient to have their details and medical history re-checked, usually by telephone, to ensure that there have been no changes to their medical or social history since the first assessment.

Summary

A pre-admission assessment helps patients focus on their surgery and find out more information on what is going to happen during the whole experience. Assessment of the patient by doctors, nurses and other health professionals is, of course, essential for ensuring an informed experience for the patient. It is also the foundation for the next stage of their surgical journey, that of actually being prepared for surgery and taken to the operating theatre. This is the focus of Chapter 6.

References

Bassett, A., 2005. Patient assessment. In: Woodhead, K., Wicker, P. (Eds.), A textbook of perioperative care. Churchill Livingstone, Edinburgh.

Beck, A., 2007. Nurse-led pre-operative assessment for elective surgical patients. Nursing Standard 21 (51), 35–38.

Carroll, A., Dowling, M., 2007. Discharge planning: communication, education and patient participation. British Journal of Nursing 16 (14), 882–886.

Crosby, D.L., Griffith, G.H., Jenkins, J.R., et al., 1972. General surgical pre-admission clinic. British Medical Journal 3 (5819), 157–159.

Department of Health, 1997. Junior doctors' hours: the new deal. DH, London.

Department of Health, 2001. National good practice on day surgery preoperative assessment. DH, London.

Department of Health, 2002. Day surgery: operational guide. DH, London.

Department of Health, 2006. The curriculum framework for the surgical care practitioner. DH, London.

Gilmartin, J., 2004. Day surgery: patients' perception of a nurse-led preadmission clinical. Journal of Clinical Nursing 13 (2), 243–250.

Goodman, H., 2010. Discharge from hospital: the importance of planning. British Journal of Cardiac Nursing 5 (6), 274–279.

Grieve, R.J., 2002. Day surgery preoperative anxiety reduction and coping strategies. British Journal of Nursing 11 (10), 670–678.

Holland, K., Hogg, C., 2010. Cultural awareness in nursing and healthcare, 2nd ed. Arnold, London.

Janke, E., Chalk, V., Kinley, H., 2002. Pre-operative assessment: setting a standard through learning. NHS Modernisation Agency, DH, London.

Johansson, K., Katajisto, J., Salanter, S., 2010. Pre-admission education in surgical rheumatology nursing: towards greater patient empowerment. Journal of Clinical Nursing 19 (21–22), 2980–2988.

Macduff, C., West, B., Harvey, S., 2001 Telemedicine in rural care. Part 2: assessing the wider issues. Nursing Standard 15 (33), 33.

National Institute for Health and Clinical Excellence, 2003. Preoperative tests. NICE, London.

NHS Modernisation Agency, 2002. National good practice guidance on pre-operative assessment for day surgery. DH, London.

NHS Scotland, 2008. The national framework for service change in NHS Scotland – elective care action team, final report. NHS Scotland, Edinburgh.

Nursing and Midwifery Council, 2010. Standards for pre-registration nursing education. NMC, London.

Oakley, M., Bratchell, J., 2010. Preoperative assessment. In: Pudner, R. (Ed.), Nursing the surgical patient, 3rd ed. Baillière Tindall, Edinburgh: 3–13.

Pritchard, M.J., 2009. Managing anxiety in the elective surgical patient. British Journal of Nursing 18 (7), 416–419.

Royal College of Nursing, 2006. Meeting the health needs of people with learning disabilities. RCN, London.

Scottish Executive, 2005. Building a health service fit for the future. The Scottish Government, Edinburgh.

Shepperd, S., McClaran, J., Phillips, C.O., et al., 2010. Discharge planning from hospital to home. Cochrane Database of Systematic Reviews (1) doi:10.1002/14651858.CD000313.pub3.

Smith, L., Callery, P., 2005. Children's accounts of their preoperative information needs. Journal of Clinical Nursing 14 (2), 230–238.

Further reading

Digner, M., 2007. At your convenience: preoperative assessment by telephone. Journal of Perioperative Practice 17 (7), 294–301.

Harvey, S., 2001. Telemedicine in rural care. Part 1: developing and evaluating a nurse-led initiative. Nursing Standard 15 (32), 33.

Hughes, S.J., Mardell, A., 2009. Oxford handbook of perioperative practice. Oxford University Press, Oxford.

Oakley, M., Bratchell, J., 2010. Preoperative assessment. In: Pudner, R. (Ed.), Nursing the surgical patient, 3rd ed. Baillière Tindall, Edinburgh.

Simmons, M., 1998. Preoperative skin preparation. Professional Nurse 13 (7), 446–447.

Wicker, P., O'Neill, J., 2010. Caring for the perioperative patient, 2nd ed. Wiley-Blackwell, Oxford.

Woodhead, K., Wicker, P., 2005. A textbook of perioperative care. Churchill Livingstone, Edinburgh.

Websites

The NICE website offers national guidance on preoperative tests: http://www.nice.org.uk/Guidance/CG3 (accessed December 2011).

The Association for Perioperative Practice (AfPP) began life as the National Association of Theatre Nurses in 1964. It is a charity providing education and support to theatre nurses, operating department practitioners and all those working in and around operating departments: http://www.afpp.org.uk (accessed December 2011).

A website links directly to the NICE guidelines on the use of preoperative tests for elective surgery: http://www.nice.org.uk/nicemedia/pdf/Preop_Fullguideline.pdf (accessed May 2011).

The NHS Choices website focuses on a preoperative assessment talk for patients by a nurse: http://www.nhs.uk/video/pages/pre-operativeassessments.aspx?searchtype=Tag&searchterm=Liver_Digestion__Bowel_Rectum (accessed December 2011).

The website of the NHS Institute for Innovation and Improvement: http://www.institute.nhs.uk/quality_and_service_improvement_tools/quality_and_service_improvement_tools/discharge_planning.html (accessed December 2011).

6

Preparation of the patient for surgery: the hospital experience

CHAPTER AIMS

- To explore the continuity of care from a pre-admission assessment to being admitted for surgery
- To explore the care delivery after admission to hospital and being prepared for the operating theatre
- To determine all the preoperative procedures and protocols required to ensure a safe transfer from ward to anaesthetic room and operating theatre
- To consider the actual and potential problems that patients may experience prior to undergoing surgery

Introduction

Chapter 5 introduced you to what happens prior to patients being admitted for surgery, including pre-admission assessment and identifying what may be required in readiness for their discharge home from hospital. This chapter focuses on what happens when someone actually enters the hospital, undergoes admission to the ward or unit where they are to stay prior to and after surgery and their preparation prior to surgery. For most patients and their families, this can be a very stressful time, and even more so if their admission to hospital has been an emergency.

Care of the patient on admission to hospital

Admission to hospital is part of the 'perioperative' period of care (i.e. three phases of preoperative, intraoperative and postoperative) (Pudner 2010). The admission may be planned, with most patients having had a preoperative assessment to ensure specific needs or problems are identified, stress is reduced by information sharing and, in these times, to reduce the risk of a hospital-acquired infection (Pudner 2010:3). Another term for this is 'elective' surgery. It may also be an admission for 'emergency' surgery which has not been planned.

Read Gilmour's (2010) explanation in Box 6.1 before considering the nursing care aspect of the preoperative period.

So what role does the nurse play in a planned admission?

Activity

If this is your first or second surgical placement, find out prior to your first week what kind of surgical procedures are identified as planned or 'elective'. Your university placement learning website may offer some information but you may also need to visit the placement, introducing yourself to staff at the same time. Make a list in your notebook and find out as much as you can about the underlying pathophysiology (i.e. what has gone wrong with the body's normal physiology) and what procedures the surgeon is likely to undertake. (See Further Reading for some medical textbooks illustrating surgical procedures, and websites for further examples.)

Planned admission

Patients may undergo planned surgery on a day care basis, a short stay basis or they may stay longer in hospital. It is important to consider the impact of introducing a 'surgical' journey which can now take place in a single day. In the past, most surgical procedures required patients to stay in for longer. The parallel developments in surgical techniques and technology have revolutionised care and the kinds of experiences students now experience in clinical practice placements.

It should be noted, however, that changes to length of stay in hospital have created different expectations of nurses who work in a community setting. If your placement is in a community setting, you will meet patients who now require a higher level of nursing care or observation postoperatively, including support for their carer at this time. In the past patients would stay in hospital for nurses to observe for postoperative complications such as wound infection and removal of sutures. This has become more the responsibility of the community team.

Box 6.1 Elective or emergency surgery (Gilmour 2010:18)

Elective surgery aims to be performed when the patient is in optimal health but before the surgery affects the quality and threatens their life: e.g. an inguinal hernia can become life-threatening if the bowel becomes obstructed within the sac. Clinicians decide if a planned procedure is urgent or can be arranged at a time convenient for the surgeon and patient (Phillips 2004).

Emergency surgery may be as a result of trauma or an accident, gastrointestinal obstruction or from perforated viscera. The injury may be immediately life-threatening, and therefore the procedure will be carried out with 1–2 hours from admission. Other emergencies may require procedures within 24–48 hours following the injury, but in both instances the preoperative time for preparing the patient is significantly reduced and changes to the patient's condition occur rapidly. Information may be limited; the perioperative nurse must be prepared for any event or occurrence, and therefore communication within the perioperative team is essential to coordinate the delivery of safe patient care during this potentially traumatic period (MacDonald 2005).

Care of the patient within 12 hours of being prepared for surgery

Most patients arrive at hospital with a relative or friend. Some patients who have been in hospital a long time ago may expect to be asked to change into their pyjamas, slippers and dressing gown as soon as they arrive! This is no longer always the case, unless of course they may have to undergo tests or examinations as soon as they arrive in the ward. It is important to remember, however, that some elderly patients faced with a hospital stay may have purchased new nightclothes to be a patient – they may not feel that they are 'properly ill' or a 'proper patient' unless they are dressed for bed. Being sensitive to their needs is important.

Instructions sent to patients by the hospital inform them of what clothes to bring in and other important information (see Box 6.2 for examples). Knowing this information is helpful during the assessment of a patient on admission to hospital.

Box 6.2 Key patient information for hospital admission for surgery

Pre-arrival

Patients should complete any documentation sent pre-admission to take with them – this may include special dietary needs and any recent infections.

Patients may have been advised to give up smoking, lose weight or have other health problems checked for stability, for example diabetes.

Clothing and personal items: information on what to bring, such as pyjamas or nightdress, dressing gown, slippers, personal toiletries. If a longer stay is possible, patients should bring some casual clothes for their time of recuperation pre-discharge home. If having knee or hip surgery, for example, they could also be asked to bring shorts or track suit type clothes plus comfortable supportive shoes for wearing during postoperative physiotherapy sessions.

Medications: it is very important that patients bring *all* their medications (plus any original information).

Valuables: patients are advised not to bring valuables or large sums of money if at all possible.

Mobile phones and any electrical equipment: these may interfere with hospital equipment and their use may be restricted in key areas.

On arrival

If arriving on the day of surgery or the day before, patients will be admitted by a nurse and all information about them checked, especially their understanding of the impending surgery. Contact details are obtained and a patient identity bracelet must be worn at all times during the stay.

The day before: patients may be allowed to eat and drink as normal until told otherwise and depending on the type of surgery.

Continued

Box 6.2 Key patient information for hospital admission for surgery—cont'd

The same day: patients may not be allowed to eat for at least 6 hours prior to surgery and may only drink clear fluids up to 2 hours preoperatively. Again this is dependent on the type of surgery.

Patients should be informed about the surgery, possible side effects such as nausea/vomiting, pain and pain control, specific postoperative exercises, avoiding deep vein thrombosis and advice on smoking. Depending on the type of surgery, there may be further information.

Going to the operating theatre

Informed consent: the patient will need to understand the nature of their surgery and sign a consent form either in the pre-admission assessment or on admission following a visit by the anaesthetist or consultant surgeon. It is important to check this.

The anaesthetic procedure should be explained to the patient as well as what will happen in the operating theatre and why they may get pain postoperatively. The effects of anaesthesia should also be explained, especially nausea and why the throat may be sore post-operatively after having an endotracheal tube in place during the anaesthetic.

Their named nurse and/or student may accompany patients to the operating theatre along with theatre personnel.

After surgery

A brief explanation of what happens in the operating theatre, who is present and what to expect postoperatively on the ward may be included. The effects of surgery and anaesthesia should be explained briefly as well.

Going home

Going home from hospital following surgery will already have been discussed on admission – it is essential that patients consider this before surgery and discuss with the nurse on admission any issues relating to home care and, possibly, home care facilities and requirements on discharge home. Some types of surgery will have specific going home instructions, e.g. after removal of part of the bowel, patients will be advised how to manage dietary intake and stoma care (if they have one).

✔ **Tip**

When you begin your placement experience, find out what hospital policies are in place with regards to patients admitted for surgery and, in particular, any that directly involve the role of the nurse and other healthcare professionals. Discuss how to obtain access to these with your mentor.

Find out as much information as you can about patient information leaflets available for patients on your ward so that you are prepared to answer their questions.

☑ **Tip**

A NHS Choices video explains how patients can prepare for admission to hospital:
http://www.nhs.uk/Video/Pages/Preparingforhospital.aspx (accessed December 2011).

◐ **Activity**

Here are some other approaches linked to care delivery that you may come across in practice or in your reading. Identify their meaning and make some notes. These are often used as part of student assignments involving delivery of patient care (see Appendix 1 at the end of this chapter for brief notes on each):

- Named nurse.
- Primary nursing.
- Team nursing.
- Patient allocation.
- Task allocation.

Depending on the ward/unit, patients may be allocated a 'named nurse' who will coordinate the delivery of care from admission to discharge home. The named nurse approach to care delivery is one of many terms you will come across during your learning in practice and in theory.

Once a patient has been shown to his or her bed and shown around the ward/unit so that they are familiar with bathroom facilities and the day room, the nurse can introduce them to other patients if appropriate. If the patient is going to theatre on the same day they are admitted to hospital, they will not have much time to communicate with others but will have to undergo preoperative preparation by the nurse.

It is important for relatives or carers to know visiting times or the best time to phone to find out how the patient is, as people accompanying patients on arrival soon have to leave. Even prior to the formal patient assessment, it is important to determine any special and immediate needs of patients or anything relatives might wish to let the nurses know about. One example could be whether the patient requires a translator or not and whether they speak or read English. During the assessment process, it is essential that all patients are able to understand what is being asked of them or what they may be required to sign. It may be that someone attending with the patient is required to stay with them until they actually leave the ward to go to the operating theatre.

◐ **Activity**

Imagine you are a student nurse on placement in a female general surgical ward. Your mentor has asked if you would like to assist her in admitting a woman to the ward who is to go to theatre later that afternoon for a thyroidectomy. She has already attended a pre-admission clinic 2 weeks previously and is likely to have to stay in hospital for at least 2 days postoperatively. You agree to work with your mentor as this

Continued

is one of the learning goals you have set yourself on this placement. You also agree with your mentor that this would be an excellent opportunity to follow a patient's journey and care until she is discharged from hospital. Your mentor has agreement from the theatre team for you to attend the surgery and immediate postoperative care with the patient in the recovery ward.

1. What do you think is essential to know prior to meeting the patient and undertaking the admission assessment?
2. What approach to assessment is the mentor likely to consider to help her make a full assessment of the patient?
3. As a student nurse, what will be your priority within the team to discuss with the patient?
4. What specific potential problems is this patient at risk of developing postoperatively and what observations will nurses be undertaking to detect them?

Some general issues to consider

It is essential to know the patient's pre-admission assessment information, which should include the physiological, psychological and social needs of the patient, and any information which could be important for her wellbeing during and after her operation. Familiarising yourself with this information is very important in order to ensure that any sensitive issues are noted as well as important health ones.

1. A key check with the patient is to ensure that she has followed the specific pre-admission instructions she was given with regards to preoperative fasting. The Royal College of Nursing (RCN) guideline on perioperative fasting in adults and children, which is based on a range of evidence, recommends for adults: 'Intake of water up to 2 hours before induction of anaesthesia and a minimum preoperative fasting time of 6 hours for food (solids, milk and milk-containing drinks' (RCN 2005:4).

    Contact details of relatives or other carers are important.

2. Your mentor will use the assessment document and procedure used in your particular placement. This may use a standard care plan, an integrated care pathway document, an electronic assessment tool and/or a nursing model/framework for assessment (e.g. the Roper, Logan and Tierney model of nursing (Holland et al 2008)). Regardless of how the assessment is documented, it is important to consider the nursing process of assessment, planning, implementing and evaluating in devising both the assessment stage and the care plan generally. Your mentor will also ensure that the patient has signed the consent form for surgery and that she fully understands the surgery to be undertaken.

3. As a student, it is important to ensure that the patient is aware that you are a student nurse and a team member. It is also important to let her know that you will be going with her to the operating theatre, anaesthetic room and staying with her until she is back on the ward again. Ensuring she is happy with this arrangement can be discussed with your mentor.

4. Postoperative problems and detection: in the immediate postoperative period, there are general postoperative

problems that can occur for any patient who has undergone an anaesthetic and surgical intervention that nurses have to be alert to. Examples are shock, pain, nausea or difficulty breathing. For someone who has had a thyroidectomy, there are specific potential ones such as damage to the laryngeal nerve, a haematoma pressing on the trachea, thyroid crisis, risk of tetany (Refer to Ch. 13 in Pudner (2010) for an excellent outline of the total nursing care of patients using the Roper, Logan and Tierney model of nursing).

With regards to the exercises above, see also Ch. 5 in this book for more general comments on pre-operative assessment.

Immediate preoperative care of the patient prior to surgery

Once a patient has been assessed and any immediate needs identified, they will need to undergo preparation for transfer to the operating theatre.

There are a number of books which consider this (see Further Reading), so here we consider the main issues while some others are considered in earlier chapters.

Depending on the kind of surgical intervention the patient is having, there are both general and specific preoperative preparation needs. For example, someone going for an operation involving their hip joint will need different considerations to someone undergoing surgery on their eyes. Let us look at what you will be involved in as general preoperative preparation.

Depending on where your main placement is in the perioperative period and also the kind of surgery that takes place there, you will meet patients at a number of different stages. Understanding the whole pathway of care is essential for understanding the experience patients undergo. For example, if you are caring for a patient in a ward, being able to explain why they may feel bruised or have 'aches and pains' in places they didn't expect – as a result of their positioning on the operating table for a period of time – will help to allay their fears.

A brief introduction is offered here together with further reading for you to pursue prior to commencement of your placement.

General preparation
Psychological preparation
We use the term 'psychological' here to outline some of the reassuring activities you can undertake regarding the impending surgery, as opposed to the physical preparation activities that you are required to undertake.

> **⬛ Activity**
>
> Consider the example given in Box 6.3 and think about what could have helped this patient to be less anxious.
>
> Read the articles by Leinonen and Leino-Kilpi (1999), Mitchell (2000) and Pritchard (2009) (see References) to help you to provide an evidence-based response for reducing preoperative anxiety.

Physical preparation
As well as managing potential anxiety and worries preoperatively, there are specific preparation requirements that nurses and others have to undertake. It is not possible to offer specific preoperative preparation for all types of surgery here, so we mainly focus on the general but give some specific examples. It is important that you read about the kinds of surgery you will encounter on your clinical placement and focus on understanding both general and specific preoperative preparation of patients, why they must take place and the possible outcomes if they are not

---

Box 6.3 Practice example: preoperative preparation of a patient going to theatre

Mrs Peters, a 45-year-old woman, was admitted to hospital for a hysterectomy. Her initial pre-admission assessment showed that the outcome of this surgery had been discussed with her, and the possibility that the gynaecologist would also have to remove both her ovaries, thus causing an early menopause. Some literature had been given to her to read about this by the pre-admission assessment nurse, but she hadn't fully understood the implications of this. She had had no time to discuss it with anyone as she was admitted for surgery 2 weeks after the assessment. She signed the consent form at this time as well, thinking she was clear about her surgery.

On admission to the ward, the nurse (your mentor) undertook a further assessment of her immediate preoperative needs and this worry and anxiety about not having her ovaries after the surgery was highlighted. She made every attempt to reassure the patient and contacted the consultant and his team but none had been available to come to the ward to talk to her.

The pre-surgery physical preparation had to continue despite her concerns in order to ensure she would be ready when it was her turn to go to theatre. She was still anxious when you and your mentor took her to the operating theatre/anaesthetic room.

---

undertaken. It is also important to adopt an evidence-based approach to nursing practice (Holland 2010). The main physical preparations to consider are:

Preoperative fasting Patients can normally have clear fluids up to 2 hours preoperatively and solid food/milky drinks up to 6 hours preoperatively (RCN 2005), but this depends very much on the nature of the surgery to be undertaken. For example, patients undergoing major bowel surgery will have more intensive preoperative preparation than someone undergoing surgery for removal of varicose veins.

Preoperative fasting is important to 'ensure safety during induction of general anaesthesia by preventing inhalation of acid stomach contents into the lungs when the gag reflex is lost' (Amos & Waugh 2007:686) (see Chs 7 and 8 for further explanation).

In terms of your role in the preoperative preparation of a patient who is not allowed

---

⟲ Activity

Find out about the care of a patient with diabetes who is undergoing surgery.

Imagine you are the named nurse (supervised by your mentor) for a patient with diabetes who is to undergo major surgery, a below-the-knee amputation. Make a plan of his preoperative care needs and how you will manage his care relating to the stabilisation of his diabetes during the perioperative period.

An excellent resource for undertaking this exercise is the NHS Diabetes website: http://www.diabetes.nhs.uk (accessed December 2011). Search for 'Management of adults with diabetes undergoing surgery and elective procedures: improving standards' (NHS 2011) to download the pdf.

fluids, you can ensure that the water jug is not left on the patient's bedside table. In many hospitals, you will find a sign above the patient's bed saying 'nil by mouth', meaning they must have nothing to drink or eat. It is also important to note that some patients are at risk when they are unable to eat or drink: in particular, patients who are diabetic and insulin dependent. They will have their normal routine disturbed by the lack of food and drink, and may have intravenous fluid and nourishment, intensive monitoring of their glucose levels and linked insulin dosage (sliding scale of insulin) during the whole of the perioperative period.

Bowel preparation Preparation of the bowel prior to surgery, in particular abdominal surgery, is important for the following reasons (Amos & Waugh 2007:688):

- *Defecation during anaesthesia.*
- *Faecal contamination during surgery, particularly for surgery on the gastrointestinal tract.*
- *Postoperative stress on the wound.*
- *Postoperative discomfort or constipation due to a full rectum.*

Patients may be given laxatives to take prior to coming into hospital as part of their bowel preparation, especially if going to the operating theatre not long after admission. Patients who are admitted the day before surgery and require more extensive preparation may be given oral and/or bowel laxatives to aid the process.

Skin preparation (including hair removal) Preoperative skin care is undertaken at two levels: cleaning the skin itself and removing body hair from the surgical site (Amos & Waugh 2007). If a patient has to self-prepare prior to admission for immediate surgery, they are advised '*to have a bath or shower to remove dirt and microbes from the skin and to wash their hair, because this can act as a reservoir for bacteria* (Simmons 1998)' (Scott et al 2007).

If the patient is already in hospital, they will require a similar preparation and as part of the immediate preoperative preparation will be given a clean theatre gown to wear and required to remove all clothing as necessary. Scott et al (2007) state that the evidence is inconclusive with regards to removal of body hair – one view is that it should be removed because hair harbours bacteria which could be introduced into the wound, and the other view is that getting rid of hair increases the risk of infection by reducing the body's natural defence mechanisms.

It is important to understand that removing body hair is not allowed in some cultures, for example the Sikh religion. This would be an issue for negotiation with the patient and possibly the Sikh chaplain (see http://www.sikhchaplaincy.org.uk/Booklet.pdf (accessed December 2011)).

🔖 Activity

> Read the articles by Dean and Fawcett (2002), Murkin (2009) and the RCN (2005) (see References) which are relevant to these areas of preoperative preparation. Make notes on the key points of the underpinning evidence base to nursing actions in each case.

Final preoperative preparation of the patient (identified in Amos & Waugh 2007)

The key actions in brief are:

Emptying the bladder
It is important that patients go to the toilet immediately prior to going to theatre, to ensure they do not become incontinent during surgery (if there is a long delay, they may need to go again). '*For patients having extensive pelvic surgery and an epidural or spinal anaesthesia, a urinary catheter is passed (usually in theatre) to ensure that the bladder remains empty and that urinary output*

can be measured accurately postoperatively' (Amos & Waugh 2007:691).

Theatre clothing As noted earlier, patients are required to put on a clean operating theatre gown. Antiembolic stockings may also be required (and patients need to wear the right size).

Activity

Find out about the policy on your placement with regards to wearing antiembolic stockings and ask your mentor to show you how to measure and put these on a patient prior to surgery.

The information on the NHS Choices website will help you with the National Institute for Health and Clinical Excellence (NICE) evidence base for wearing antiembolic stockings: http://www.nhs.uk/chq/Pages/2609. aspx?CategoryID=69&SubCategoryID =692 (accessed December 2011).

Removal of cosmetics, jewellery and prostheses All cosmetics must be removed so that any pallor can be seen and, importantly, nail varnish must be removed to ensure any signs of cyanosis can be seen. Jewellery is also removed but, if requested, a wedding ring can be kept on and taped securely. Any jewellery removed is either sent home with relatives or kept in a hospital safe, depending on hospital policy. Removal of metal objects prevents contact burns from diathermy equipment or damage to the patient if caught on a piece of equipment (Amos & Waugh 2007).

Allergies Allergies should be checked again as patients may have forgotten to mention these if worried about their impending surgery. Some allergies can be caused by skin preparation liquids used in theatre.

Identity bands Patients must wear these on admission as they are vital to ensure that the right patient goes to the operating theatre. They are very important when a patient is unable to communicate effectively as a result of anaesthesia.

Premedication If a patient has been admitted for day surgery, premedication is not normally used. Other patients may receive a light sedative to reduce anxiety, and some are also *'given an anticholinergic drug, such as hyoscine, to reduce oral and bronchial secretions and vagal overactivity'* (Amos and Waugh 2007) prior to an anaesthetic and to reduce incidence of inhalation when the gag reflex is lost.

Final preoperative checks

Prior to a patient being transported to the operating theatre, it is important to check again that all necessary activities have been undertaken and a broad checklist is provided in Figure 6.1.

Transfer of the patient from the ward to the operating theatre

Actually leaving the ward area and being transported on a trolley, or sometimes on their own hospital bed, with unfamiliar people can be one of the most frightening and stressful experiences for patients. Oakley and Pudner (2010:47) state that *'the benefits of reducing anxiety in the surgical patient are not disputed; if a patient is nervous they may experience more pain following surgery, as increased anxiety leads to increased muscle tension, which in turn leads to increased pain as well as to an increase in blood pressure'*.

If you are looking after patients who are going to theatre, you may have planned with your mentor to be with a patient during the whole perioperative period. If this is a learning goal, then accompanying the patient from the ward to the operating theatre and anaesthetic room is absolutely essential. It also means that the patient has someone they know with them during this anxious time who will also be with them when they wake up from the anaesthetic.

We have considered the journey of patients who have a planned admission for surgery. We now consider the emergency admission of a patient for surgery.

NAME:			Consultant		
Date of birth:					
Unit number:					
Weight:					

Please tick	Yes	No	Please tick	Yes	No
Allergies, state:			Case notes including latest laboratory results		
Consent form signed			X-rays		
Identiband on wrist/ankle			Fluid balance chart		
Operation site identified			Medicine records		
Hair removed from operation site			Nursing notes		
Make up/nail varnish removed			Manual handling risk assessment form completed and with records		
Fasted			Antiembolism stockings applied		
Premedication given			Bladder emptied/Catheterized		
EMLA cream applied			Jewellery removed/taped		
Dentures removed			Body piercings and other metal objects removed		
Hearing aid in situ			Modesty pants		
Spectacles with patient			Menstruating Pad/Tampon in situ		
Contact lenses removed			Crowns/loose teeth present, if yes, where?		
Other prosthesis in situ (state):			Pressure ulcer risk assessment score		

Ward Nurse: Printed Name	Signature
Theatre Nurse: Printed Name	Signature

Fig 6.1 Preoperative checklist

Activity

Discuss with your mentor a plan for total patient care and experiencing the patient pathway throughout the perioperative period. Explain it to the patient and gain their permission to be with them and present during their surgery. If it is major surgery, make sure you eat and drink beforehand, as standing in the operating theatre for a long time on an empty stomach, in a gown, mask and hat, can be extremely uncomfortable and may cause you to faint. If you feel faint (see later chapters), it is important that you leave the operating theatre immediately.

When you arrive at the operating theatre, you will 'hand over' the patient to the anaesthetic nurse or operating department assistant. Prior to your visit, it is important that everyone is aware you will be staying to observe the surgery and be with the patient in the postoperative recovery area.

Emergency admission

In many instances, a patient who is considered an emergency admission may be transferred immediately to the operating theatre from the accident and emergency department. The first time you meet them may be during your operating theatre placement or when they return to the ward where you are on a surgical placement.

Some patients, however, may need to be stabilised first and may be admitted to a short-stay emergency care ward or a surgical ward prior to their surgery. For example, an elderly lady who has fallen in the street and fractured her femur may be taken to the orthopaedic ward prior to surgery.

Emergency surgery patients may undergo further tests and be under very close observation and monitoring. If they are conscious, they will be very anxious, and your role in their care involves making sure they are kept informed as appropriate about what is happening to them. Their family/relatives may not be aware of their admission and this may be dealt with by the police or by the senior ward staff.

Information about the general health of emergency surgical patients may be unknown, especially if they are not fully aware of what is happening to them. Tests to see if they are diabetic or not, for example, will be vital.

Some patients carry vital health information with them as well as information about medications such as steroids. They may also carry a donor card.

How critical a patient is will determine when they are taken to the operating theatre.

Summary

This chapter provided a brief overview of the care of the patient who is to undergo surgery. There have been major advances in surgical techniques over the past 20 years, with patients requiring less time in hospital for major surgery. Day surgery is now common and other patients may go home more quickly than an agreed stay in hospital. If your placement is in a surgical unit, you will have an opportunity to engage in one-to-one care of individual patients during their journey. You will also learn about different types of surgery and the various preparations required in order to manage actual and potential postoperative problems likely to be encountered. Chapter 7 explores another stage in the patient journey: the anaesthetic room.

References

Amos, A., Waugh, A., 2007. Caring for the person having surgery. In: Brooker, C., Waugh, A. (Eds.), Foundations of nursing practice. Mosby, Edinburgh: 681–702.

Dean, A., Fawcett, T., 2002. Nurses' use of evidence in pre-operative fasting. Nursing Standard Art and Science 17 (12), 33–37.

Gilmour, D., 2010. Perioperative care. In: Pudner, R. (Ed.), Nursing the surgical patient, 3rd ed. Baillière Tindall, Edinburgh.

Holland, K., 2010. Evidence-based practice and its implementation in nursing. In: Holland, K., Rees, C. (Eds.), Nursing: evidence-based practice skills. Oxford University Press, Oxford: 197–221.

Holland, K., Jenkins, J., Solomon, J., Whittam, S., 2008. Applying the Roper, Logan and Tierney model in practice. Churchill Livingstone, Edinburgh.

Leinonen, T., Leino-Kilpi, H., 1999. Research in peri-operative nursing care. Journal of Clinical Nursing 8 (2), 123–138.

Mitchell, M., 2000. Anxiety management: a distinct nursing role in day surgery. Ambulatory Surgery 8 (3), 119–127.

Murkin, C., 2009. Pre-operative antiseptic skin preparation. British Journal of Nursing 18 (11), 665–669.

Oakley, M., Pudner, R., 2010. Preoperative stress and anxiety in the surgical patient.

In: Pudner, R. (Ed.), Nursing the surgical patient, third ed. Baillière Tindall, Edinburgh: 45–51.

Pritchard, M.J., 2009. Managing anxiety in the elective surgical patient. British Journal of Nursing 18 (7), 416–419.

Pudner, R. (Ed.), 2010. Nursing the surgical patient. Baillière Tindall, Edinburgh.

Royal College of Nursing, 2005. Perioperative fasting in adults and children: an RCN guideline for the multidisciplinary team. Clinical Practice Guidelines Series. RCN, London.

Scott, C., McArthur-Rouse, F.J., McLean, J., 2007. Pre-operative assessment and preparation. In: McArthur-Rouse, F., Prosser, S. (Eds.), Assessing and managing the acutely ill adult surgical patient. Blackwell, Oxford: 3–16.

Shebini, N., Aggarwal, R., Gandhi, A., 2008. Improved patient awareness of named nursing through audit. Nursing Times 104 (21), 30–31.

Simmons, M., 1998. Preoperative skin preparation. Professional Nurse 13, 447.

Further reading

Gibson, C., 2006. The patient facing surgery. In: Alexander, M., Fawcett, J.N., Runciman, P.J. (Eds.), Nursing practice, the hospital and home: the adult. Churchill Livingstone, Edinburgh: 901–943.

Royal College of Nursing, 2008. Defending dignity: challenges and opportunities for nursing. Online. Available at: www.rcn.org.uk/__data/assets/pdf_file/0011/166655/003257.pdf (accessed December 2011).

Websites

NHS Choices videos – an excellent site for listening to patient stories of their health experiences, including surgical procedures: http://www.nhs.uk/video/pages/MediaLibrary.aspx (accessed April 2011).

The Royal College of Surgeons website – very informative for patient information pre- and post-surgery for adults and children: http://www.rcseng.ac.uk/patient_information (accessed April 2011).

NHS Scotland Clinical Governance: http://www.clinicalgovernance.scot.nhs.uk/ (accessed December 2011).

An NHS website explaining aspects of clinical governance and patient care, plus a number of excellent links to other resources: http://nhslocal.nhs.uk/our-nhs/hospital-care (accessed April 2011).

Pre- and postoperative care after bowel surgery – a two-part video from a UK hospital in partnership with Coloplast UK for prospective patients to be admitted to hospital. It uses 'lay' language that service users can understand without all the technical 'jargon': http://www.youtube.com/watch?v=flgO6mUaHbM (accessed December 2011).

Appendix 1 Brief meaning of nursing care approaches

1. **Named nurse:** this term is used mainly in the UK and, according to some authors, has been adopted to mean the same in terms of care delivery as primary nursing has in the USA. The patient is allocated a named nurse on admission to hospital, and Shebini et al (2008) cite the Scottish Office (1992) definition as: *'A registered nurse, midwife or health visitor who is responsible for assessing, planning, implementing, evaluating and coordinating patient care on an individual basis with a patient or a caseload of patients from admission/transfer/discharge'.*

Continued

Appendix 1 Brief meaning of nursing care approaches—cont'd

2. **Primary nursing:** this is a system where the total care of an individual patient and his/her family is the responsibility of one nurse – the primary nurse. They are accountable for the overall care and have the authority to make decisions as the 'leader' of the care provided. They are possibly the primary nurse for a small group of patients, delivering individualised and patient-centred care for the whole of their contact with the patient. They are supported by secondary nurses who carry out the care planned by the primary nurse, even when the primary nurse is not available due to off-duty rotas, for example. Some secondary nurses are also primary nurses for their own patients, and decision making and leadership is therefore an integral part of the primary nursing approach to care delivery. The original philosophy of primary nursing is described in a YouTube clip by Professor Marie Manthey (who led a project about the development of this approach and has since become known as the originator of it internationally): http://www.encyclopedia.com/video/kr7t8E5MMoM-primary-nursing-short-story-by.aspx (accessed December 2011).

3. **Team nursing:** this is a system of providing care as a group of healthcare workers (registered and non-registered) where there is a nominated team leader, normally a qualified nurse. The team leader is responsible for leading the team's work and also for taking overall responsibility for the planning, delivery and evaluation of the care given. The team leader normally agrees the assignment of care duties with the team and reports directly to the ward manager/sister or person in charge. Team nursing enables development of leadership and management skills, but individual members of the team remain individually accountable and/or responsible for the care they give.

4. **Patient allocation:** this is a system where each nurse is allocated a small group of patients to deliver care to, usually on a shift-by-shift or day rota basis. It is not as defined as team nursing where the team leader's role is normally a set one and the team leader's name is identified on the staff rota list. It allows for an opportunity, in particular, for student nurses to take responsibility for a small group to patients under the guidance and supervision of their mentors, learning not only about the delivery of quality care but also a range of skills such as those adopted by a team leader (e.g. delegation skills, working with others, communication and accountability).

5. **Task allocation:** this is a very 'traditional' method of care delivery and is focused not on the individual patient and their care but on the task required in their care. For example, a member of staff could be allocated to take every patient's temperature, pulse and respiration, another to take everyone's blood pressure and another could be tasked with 'doing the medicines or medicine round'. Task allocation often leads to a hierarchy of tasks and who does them, with less junior staff being delegated those which are considered 'mundane' or less important than others.

It is important to note that in many care delivery settings, a combination of these approaches can be found working very well in accordance with patients' needs as well as ensuring that quality care is delivered.

Preparation for and undergoing an anaesthetic prior to surgery

CHAPTER AIMS

- To consider the nurse's role in the anaesthetic room
- To provide an overview of modern anaesthetic practices
- To provide an introduction to the commonest types of anaesthesia
- To describe the broad principles of patient care related to the specific anaesthetic administered

Introduction

The field of anaesthetics is vast and complex. This chapter can only aim to give a brief insight into this complex area of service provision. There are many good texts that you can use to gain more in-depth knowledge on particular aspects which we only touch on. Equally, the experience and expertise of the anaesthetic team are a good source for you to gain further knowledge about caring for the patient who is about to undergo surgery.

At the end of Chapter 6, a patient was transferred to the operating theatre from the ward accompanied by a nurse. The patient is then taken into the anaesthetic room and handed over from the ward nurse to either the anaesthetic nurse or operating

department practitioner (ODP). This is a very vulnerable time for patients and, especially if they have never experienced an anaesthetic before, they will rely very much on the security of the familiar nurse from the ward. This may well be you.

Transfer of the patient to the anaesthetic room

If the patient is to undergo major surgery, they will be taken to the anaesthetic room either on their bed, a theatre trolley or, if day surgery, a wheelchair or on foot (Gilmour 2010). Here they will meet new staff, in particular the anaesthetist, the anaesthetic nurse or operating department practitioner. They all have roles to play in caring for the patient and ensuring safe practice in the anaesthetic room (see Box 7.1 for the main functions of staff providing anaesthetic assistance).

In the handover period between ward staff and anaesthetic room staff, it is important that all details about the patient, their surgery and consent form have been checked – this may take place outside the immediate anaesthetic room, in the 'clean area' beyond the doors to the main operating theatre suite.

The patient must be treated with respect and dignity at all times. Any cultural or religious needs must be taken into account during this time and reassurance given about such issues as modesty, body fluids and skin

---

Box 7.1 Main functions of staff providing anaesthetic assistance

Provision of a safe environment

- *Preparing equipment, medicines and fluids.*
- *Checking monitors and apparatus.*
- *Ensuring adequate stock.*
- *Ensuring a clean environment and equipment.*

Administrative functions

- *Arranging to send for the patient from the ward/clinic.*
- *Ensuring correct patient for correct procedure.*
- *Recording patient details in departmental records/database.*
- *Ensuring appropriate information accompanies the patient (case notes, results, forms, etc.).*

Communication

- *Providing the patient with an explanation and reassurance.*

- *Relaying information from the patient to the surgeon or anaesthetist.*
- *Providing a link to ensure colleagues are appropriately informed (ward, scrub team, recovery).*

Practical functions

- *Assisting with induction of anaesthesia and airway management.*
- *Assisting with local anaesthetic blocks.*
- *Assisting with the positioning of the patient.*

Expertise

- *Observing the patient's condition.*
- *Monitoring for any adverse effects of the anaesthesia.*
- *Monitoring for the maintenance of fluids and medications.*
- *Ensuring that safe systems of work are being employed at all times.*

Adapted from National Occupational Standards for Operating Department Practice (Scottish Government 2003)

Activity

If the operating theatre is your main placement (hub), it is important that you consider what you need to learn in relation to caring for patients during the handover period and also what is going to happen to the patient when they receive anaesthesia and their subsequent management.

Your mentor may already have planned an experience for you during your placement which may include more than a day in this area, working alongside the anaesthetist and others (see Appendix 1 at the end of this chapter for specific learning outcomes that can be achieved).

care as necessary (see Association for Perioperative Practice (2007) for information on respecting cultural diversity in the perioperative setting).

See Box 7.2 for a description of what the anaesthetic nurse has to manage, and identify the areas you need to learn more about. Some of the activities are identified in

---

> **Box 7.2** The role of the anaesthetic nurse
>
> *The anaesthetic nurse will, based on the information known, or relayed by the anaesthetist, prepare the anaesthetic room, anaesthetic machines and all other equipment to ensure the maintenance of a safe environment for the delivery of care during anaesthesia. This will include not only preparing the anaesthetic equipment but also applying knowledge and skills of anaesthesia related to age, medical history and surgical procedure to ensure that the patient's individual needs are being met, e.g. if the patient is elderly, additional precautions are needed when caring for their skin; if the patient has language difficulties, an interpreter may be required.*
>
> *(From Gilmour 2010:19)*

this chapter as well as resources you can access to learn more.

If you are going to spend some time in the perioperative environment of the anaesthetic room as well as caring for the patient both pre- and postoperatively, an understanding of the basics of anaesthesia is essential.

Who else is in the anaesthetic team?

The anaesthetic team includes a number of professionals, including the anaesthetic nurse as described already.

Anaesthetist

The team is led by an anaesthetist, who is a qualified doctor who has undergone further specialty training to be registered as an anaesthetist. The patient will have met the anaesthetist during their pre-admission

assessment visit and/or following their admission to hospital either for day surgery or for a longer stay. The anaesthetist will have explained what their role is and also checked a number of safety issues with the patient with regards to any long-term health problems

Activity

Watch this video on the NHS Choices website about anaesthesia and the role of the anaesthetist:
http://www.nhs.uk/conditions/ Anaesthesia/Pages/Introduction. aspx?url=Pages/What-is-it.aspx (accessed December 2011).

Make notes of key points of the process which you can further investigate when you are on your placement.
The video is also useful as it shows the actual physical environment of the operating theatre. The website also has many more short video clips of a wide range of surgical interventions from the perspective of patients and health professionals.

and medication being taken and will answer any questions they and their family might ask.

The anaesthetist ensures that patient safety is maintained during surgery, whether minor or major, and if a patient is having a general anaesthetic and is unconscious throughout the procedure, they ensure they wake up with as few problems as possible.

Operating department practitioner

Another key role in the team is that of the operating department practitioner, who provides anaesthetic assistance to the anaesthetist. The role of ODPs is multifaceted and they also contribute to the care of the patient during the actual surgery as well as during the anaesthesia. They undertake a similar period of training and education to either diploma or degree level that a student nurse does. See the NHS careers information in Box 7.3.

Definition of anaesthesia and anaesthetic

The NHS Choice website (http://www.nhs.uk/conditions/anaesthesia/Pages/Introduction.aspx (accessed May 2011) states that:

Anaesthesia means 'loss of sensation'. Medications that cause anaesthesia are called anaesthetics. Anaesthetics are used for pain relief during tests or surgical operations so that you do not feel:

- *pain*
- *touch*
- *pressure*
- *temperature.*

As seen in the NHS Choices video of the anaesthetist (see above), there are three main overarching types of anaesthesia, namely local, regional and general.

Box 7.3 NHS careers information

Working as an operating department practitioner

Operating department practitioners (ODPs) are an important part of the operating department team working with surgeons, anaesthetists and theatre nurses to help ensure every operation is as safe and effective as possible.

ODPs provide high standards of patient care and skilled support alongside medical and nursing colleagues during perioperative care. The ODP's role involves the application of theory to practice in a variety of clinical settings. The ODP therefore needs a broad knowledge and skill base, including management and communication skills, and will be involved with the assessment, delivery and evaluation of perioperative care.

Perioperative care can be divided into three interconnected phases:

- *Anaesthetic phase.*
- *Surgical phase.*
- *Recovery phase.*

The anaesthetic phase

During this phase, the ODP will:

- *assist the patient prior to surgery and provide individualised care*
- *need an ability to communicate and work effectively within a team*
- *undertake a role which will also involve many clinical skills such as the preparation of a wide range of specialist equipment and drugs. This includes anaesthetic machines, intravenous equipment and devices to safely secure the patient's airway during anaesthesia.*

The surgical phase

ODPs will participate, as part of the operative team, in a number of roles, including the 'scrubbed' role, application of aseptic technique, wound management and infection control.

Box 7.3 NHS careers information—cont'd

During this, phase ODPs will:

- *wear sterile gown and gloves and prepare all the necessary instruments and equipment for the procedure. This may involve complex machinery such as microscopes, lasers and endoscopes*
- *work alongside the surgeon, providing correct surgical instruments and materials in order to ensure safe and efficient completion of surgical procedures*
- *have a role in the promotion of health and safety and are therefore responsible for ensuring that surgical instruments, equipment and swabs are all accounted for throughout the surgical procedure*
- *undertake the circulating role, utilising communication and management skills, preparing the environment, equipment and acting as the link between the surgical team and other parts of the theatre and hospital*
- *be able to anticipate the requirements of the surgical team and to respond effectively.*

The recovery phase

During this phase, ODPs:

- *receive, assess and deliver patient care on their arrival into the recovery unit*
- *monitor the patient's physiological parameters and support them, providing appropriate interventions and treatment until the patient has recovered from the effects of the anaesthesia and/or surgery and is stable*
- *assess the patient in order to ensure they can be discharged back to a surgical ward area*
- *evaluate the care given during the perioperative phases (anaesthetics, surgery, recovery).*

(From http://www.nhscareers.nhs.uk/details/Default.aspx?Id=255 (accessed December 2011).

 Activity

To consider how the team works in the operating room and related areas access and read the article by Silen-Lipponen et al (2004) (see References).

Local anaesthesia

Local anaesthesia *'blocks the transmission of pain from a specific area of the body. Where only the sensory receptors are blocked, it is more correctly termed local analgesia'* (Gibson 2006:918).

Regional anaesthesia

'is used for larger or deeper operations where the nerves are harder to reach. Local anaesthetic is injected near the nerves in order to numb a larger area, but the patient remains conscious.' (Patient Information

Tip

Familiarise yourself with the effects of anaesthesia before you start your placement, or if you intend to include spending time in this environment as part of your insight learning days (spokes), and read Chapter 2, Gilmour (2010) (see References).

leaflet, NIHCE, accessed 25th May 2011). One type of regional anaesthesia is an epidural, which affects the lower half of the body, and is used in childbirth and also surgery where a general anaesthetic may not be advisable.

General anaesthesia
General anaesthesia is used where the patient is required to be unconscious for a period of time, sometimes for as much as 10 hours if it is a very complicated surgery. In this situation, the patient must not be able to feel anything, and this condition is *'characterised by loss of consciousness, analgesia and muscle relaxation'* (Gibson 2006:918). There are considered to be three stages to general anaesthesia:

- Stage 1: pain relief, heavy sedation and some muscle relaxation.
- Stage 2: patient loses consciousness but may *'exhibit wild movements and irrational behaviour but, with intravenous induction of anaesthesia, this stage is passed very quickly and may be more evident when the patient is recovering from anaesthesia'* (Gibson 2006:918).
- Stage 3: total muscle relaxation, loss of reflexes and consciousness, and the patient needs airways maintained. An endotracheal tube is introduced through the larynx, which is completely relaxed, and the patient's respiration is artificially maintained for the entire surgery.

Patients undergoing general anaesthetic can be in the third stage prior to leaving the anaesthetic room, and as soon as they are

Activity

It is beyond the scope of this book to explore all the drugs and procedures involved in anaesthesia. You are advised to read about the physiology of the nervous system and pain pathways and management as well as making a list of key drugs you are likely to encounter in the perioperative period. You can also ask your mentor and the operating theatre team any questions you may have. This information will help you explain to patients why they are experiencing some of the side effects of the procedures they have undergone as well as the drugs given to them.

Some of the more common side effects during the recovery period are seen in Box 7.4.

It is essential that you refresh your understanding of normal physiology of all the body systems plus some of the disordered physiology prior to your surgical placement. Surgery of any kind impacts on many different systems.

Box 7.4 Common side effects of anaesthesia

- Feeling sick or vomiting – about one in three people feel sick after an operation.
- Dizziness and feeling faint.
- Feeling cold and shivering for up to half an hour – this is possible after a general anaesthetic, or during, or after, a regional anaesthetic.
- Headache.
- Itchiness.
- Bruising and soreness.

(taken from NIHCE Patient information leaflet)

transferred into the operating room they will immediately be attached to an anaesthetic machine, which not only delivers the appropriate anaesthetic but also manages the mechanical ventilation of the patient during the operation.

Throughout the stages of general anaesthesia, it is vital that the nurse maintains communication with the patient, be it verbal or through touch. The patient must remain the focus of the procedures being carried out around them and their dignity maintained at all times. Patients are at their most vulnerable during the transition from the conscious to unconscious state. By staying with them throughout their whole experience, you will not only be able to answer their queries postoperatively but, most importantly, they will know that you have stayed with them throughout their surgery.

Your experience of the patient journey now enters its next phase of what happens in the operating theatre.

References

Association for Perioperative Practice, 2007. Respecting cultural diversity in the perioperative setting. Association for Perioperative Practice, Harrogate.

Gibson, C., 2006. The patient facing surgery. In: Alexander, M., Fawcett, J.N., Runciman, P.J. (Eds.), Nursing practice hospital and home: the adult, third ed. Churchill Livingstone, Edinburgh.

Gilmour, D., 2010. Perioperative care. In: Pudner, R. (Ed.), Nursing the surgical patient, 3rd ed. Baillière Tindall, Edinburgh: 17–34.

Scottish Government, 2003. Anaesthetic assistance: a strategy for training, recruitment and retention and the promulgating of safe practice. Online. Available at: http://www.scotland.gov. uk/Publications/2003/05/17153/21988 (accessed December 2011).

Silen-Lipponen, M., Tossavainen, K., Turunen, H., Smith, A., 2004. Learning about teamwork in operating room clinical placement. British Journal of Nursing 13 (5), 244–253.

Further reading

Eart, L., Huntington, S., 2007. The perioperative phase. In: McArthur-Rouse, F., Prosser, S. (Eds.), Assessing and managing the acutely ill adult surgical patient. Blackwell, Oxford.

Hughes, S.J., Mardell, A., 2009. Oxford handbook of perioperative practice. Oxford University Press, Oxford.

Wicker, P., O'Neill, J., 2010. Caring for the perioperative patient, second ed. Wiley-Blackwell, Oxford.

Website

NHS Choices website: http://www.nhs.uk/ conditions/anaesthetic-local/pages/ introduction.aspx (accessed December 2011).

Appendix 1

Specific learning experiences in anaesthetics: a checklist of learning outcomes

- Understand importance of communication in relieving patients' anxiety.
- Experience of managing the patient handover from ward nurse to anaesthetic practitioner.
- Ability to identify different methods of anaesthesia and the effects on patients.
- Experience management of patients' airways underpinned by principles of care and knowledge of physiology of airway management.
- Understand basic principles underpinning monitoring of patients' cardiac, respiratory and temperature control during anaesthesia.
- Ability to recognise the role of members of the multidisciplinary team and demonstrate ability to work within a team.

8

Undergoing surgery: the operating theatre experience

provided at the end of the chapter for you to explore various aspects of what you might learn about in this placement.

CHAPTER AIMS

- To develop an awareness of the operating theatre environment
- To understand the key principles of practice in the operating theatre
- To gain an insight into the patient's experience in the operating theatre
- To identify key learning needs to achieve in the operating theatre

Entering the operating theatre

The patient enters the theatre in the care of the anaesthetist and assistants, who will be responsible for their safety and wellbeing together with the rest of the surgical team until the end of the surgery and during the patient's time in the postoperative recovery room. We return to safety issues in the operating theatre later in the chapter; however, consider the following activity before your placement.

Introduction

In this chapter, we explain the basic principles of the operating theatre environment, the personnel who you will come across in the theatre during your placement learning experience and the broad principles of theatre practice and key health and safety considerations for both patients and theatre personnel. General principles of being a student in this environment are also explored. It is beyond the scope of this book to give full details of all aspects of caring for a patient in the operating theatre, and further reading material is

🔖 Activity

The World Health Organisation (WHO) has developed a number of resources to improve surgical patient safety worldwide

Take the time to explore this website: http://www.who.int/features/factfiles/safe_surgery/en/ (accessed December 2011).

Remember that when a patient has a general anaesthetic, it is important to maintain their dignity and respect and to maintain communication in some form throughout the stages of anaesthesia until they are in a sterile field, when touching them on the hand, for example, will no longer be possible. Of course, if they are having a regional anaesthetic where they will be awake during the surgery, then communication goes to the top of the list of importance in the care of the patient. Effective and caring communication is a fundamental part of nursing care and is one of the major domains in the NMC (2010) Standards and Competencies that you have to achieve to qualify as a nurse. In the new curricula, these will be found in your practice assessment documentation which you will take with you to all placements, given that your ongoing record of achievement (ORA) will be required from placement to placement (see further information on Domain 2 at http://standards.nmc-uk.org/PublishedDocuments/Standards%20for%20pre-registration%20nursing%20education%2016082010.pdf (accessed May 2011).

What does the operating theatre look like?

Television series such as Holby City and Gray's Anatomy have varying degrees of authenticity about their scenarios and context, some more dramatic than others. For most of us, that is as far as we get in terms of a visit to the operating theatre as a patient, but it is important to understand that for many of the patients in your care, this is their first experience.

Explanation of what will happen to patients when they get into the anaesthetic room and the operating theatre is an important part of reducing preoperative anxiety and if, as a student, you have this opportunity to have an 'insider' experience then you will be in a more informed position to help patients in your care.

The best way for you to see what the operating theatre looks like before your placement is to look at a visual presentation. You will see that it is a very 'high tech' area and many students experience the operating theatre, recovery ward and anaesthetic room during a critical care placement as well as a surgical placement.

Operating theatres in hospital are normally in a purpose-built unit set apart from the main corridors but within access of surgical wards and recovery areas. There are special safety and infection control requirements essential for an operating theatre which you will experience when you visit or have a placement there. Operating theatres usually come in groups together known as the operating theatre suite – the larger the hospital, the

 Activity

Discuss with your personal tutor your learning goals with regards to communication in this placement, either on the surgical ward or in the operating theatre. When you arrive on placement, discuss with your mentor what communication competencies you have to achieve in the placement, especially important at the various progression points to the next stage of your programme and journey to become a qualified nurse.

Activity

Consider the scenes in this video clip (which has been evaluated for its overall quality in informing you about the perioperative environment and nursing): http://www.youtube.com/watch?v=exAQC9Ync-0 (accessed December 2011).

What does it tell you about this important and key role for nurses? Imagine what you think it will look like and what you think you will feel in actually being in the operating theatre. When you have actually experienced it, reflect on your experience using a reflective model/framework and compare your pre-visit notes. This is an excellent reflection to write up for your learning portfolio.

more of these they need to accommodate the various surgeries that need to take place. They can also be attached to day surgery units and even in the community setting, in community hospitals for example.

Operating theatres can also be found in isolated places and war zones – the environment being a large tent rather than solid walls. Similar equipment will be found but the surgical team will have to adapt their practice accordingly.

 Activity

View some of the video clips in this chapter from the viewpoint of the general operating theatre environment to gain a pre-placement idea of what to expect.

Before considering the surgical experience for the patient in the operating theatre, we can briefly consider the team members and their roles. You already met some of them in Chapter 7.

The team in the operating theatre

The operating theatre is a highly specialised, multidisciplinary work environment. Operating theatre teams consist of professionals from at least four different specialties, namely anaesthetists, nurses, operating department practitioners and surgeons.

Anaesthetists are specialist doctors who are trained in anaesthesia (refer to Ch. 7).

Surgeons are doctors who have trained in a specific field of surgery following initial qualification and mandatory experience. Examples are orthopaedics, plastic surgery, gynaecology and cardiac surgery.

Scrub nurses are nurses who work directly with one or more surgeons while they are operating on the patient. Sometimes they are called instrument nurses or practitioners (Mitchell & Finn 2008).

Another similar role is the first assistant nurse, who has gained additional qualifications as well as experience in assisting the surgeon during surgery, and undertakes a high level of technical and assistant skills but does not actually carry out the surgery.

A **circulating nurse** is another type of operating theatre nurse who works on the perimeter of the operating room, monitoring patient care, ensuring that the room stays sterile and keeping track of instruments and sponges. The circulating nurse is a vital team member. This role in the USA is referred to as the circulator nurse.

The *AORN Journal* website describes the roles of the scrub nurse and the circulator nurse: http://www.aorn.org/CareerCenter/CareerDevelopment/RoleOfThePerioperativeNurse/ (accessed June 2011). You can see where the concept of 'scrub' comes from in relation to being 'scrubbed' and sterile for working in a sterile field alongside the surgeon.

Operating department practitioners participate as part of the team in a number of roles including the scrubbed role, circulating role and, as is mostly the case in the UK, act as the 'anaesthetic assistant' to the anaesthetist. Watch this YouTube clip for more information: http://www.youtube.com/watch?v=buKBoyt6WQs&feature=related (accessed December 2011).

The surgery

We have mentioned a number of different types of surgery, in particular day surgery and surgery requiring a longer hospital stay which could entail minimal invasive surgery or major surgery. It is beyond the scope of this book to cover all these in any detail but further reading is recommended on all of them. When you get to your main placement in perioperative care, it is up to you to find out more about the kinds of surgery that takes place in the operating theatre in each case, and the case studies in Section 3 focus in more detail on an example of each one of these to help you understand the care of the patient in the various perioperative environments.

Day surgery

Oakley (2010:35) describes day surgery as *'a specialist area of care where patients are admitted into a designated day surgery unit for minor and intermediate surgery, and discharged home the same day'*. Examples of the types of surgical intervention you will see in a day surgery operating theatre are given in Box 8.1.

Other, more major procedures can be undertaken according to the British Association of Day Surgery (Oakley 2010) but these are considered on a strict protocol and individual basis.

Box 8.1 Types of surgical intervention in a day surgery operating theatre

- Orchidopexy.
- Circumcision.
- Inguinal hernia.
- Excision of breast lump.
- Anal fissure dilation and excision.
- Haemorrhoidectomy.
- Laparoscopic cholecystectomy.
- Varicose vein stripping and ligation.
- Transurethral resection of bladder tumour.
- Excision of Dupuytren's contracture.
- Carpal tunnel decompression.
- Excision of ganglion.
- Arthroscopy.

- Bunion operations.
- Removal of metalware.
- Extraction of cataract with/without implants.
- Correction of squint.
- Myringotomy.
- Tonsillectomy.
- Submucous resection.
- Reduction of nasal fracture.
- Operation for bat ears.
- Dilatation and curettage/hysteroscopy.
- Laparoscopy.
- Termination of pregnancy.

(From The Audit Commission 'basket of 25' (Audit Commission 2001) cited in Oakley (2010:36))

Activity

Prior to your placement, identify exactly what each of the different kinds of surgery in Box 8.1 entails and make notes about each of them. After your placement is complete, check which ones you actually saw in a day surgery or other context and reflect on your experience in caring for patients in each situation.

Tip

Read the chapter by Oakley (2010) on day surgery if possible before you go to your day care surgery placement or other perioperative placements.

The articles by Mitchell (2010) and Mottram (2011) (see References) are also helpful.

Activity

Imagine you have been allocated to observe in the orthopaedic operating theatre for the day by your mentor in the surgical ward (main placement). Identify the four most common operations likely to be performed during that period of observation.

Consider what you need to know about the areas of the body being operated on. Make a list of all the anatomy and physiology you need to read up on if you are to make a contribution to the overall care of a patient in this setting. Examples you might see are:

- total hip replacement
- repair of fractured femur (shaft)
- removal of lumbar intervertebral disc
- repair of fractured tibia or fibula.

Minimal invasive surgery

Certainly in the day care unit, you will see examples of minimal invasive surgery (often called keyhole surgery) using the latest technology. Surgery such as laparoscopic cholecystectomy is an example. This type of surgery obviously causes less trauma for the patient and use of the equipment requires different skills and training to ensure safe practice by members of the surgical team.

An explanation of this can be seen on this video clip which is a news item by the BBC: http://www.youtube.com/watch?v=nbdVsGS29Fk (accessed December 2011).

Major surgery (requiring longer than a day)

As noted in previous chapters, this is surgery that cannot take place in a day care unit and requires a longer stay in hospital or is an emergency. Examples classed as major surgery normally requiring a general anaesthetic (see Ch. 7) are given in Box 8.2.

Box 8.2 Examples of major surgical interventions

Gynaecological surgery
- Hysterectomy (removal of uterus) sometimes along with a bilateral salpingo-oophorectomy (removal of both fallopian tubes and ovaries).

Colorectal surgery
- Abdominoperineal excision of rectum (removal of sigmoid colon and formation of an abdominal colostomy).

Upper gastrointestinal surgery
- Oesophagectomy (removal of oesophagus).

Orthopaedic surgery

Continued

Box 8.2 Examples of major surgical interventions—cont'd

■ Total hip replacement (arthroplasty) (replacement of both head of femur and acetabulum).

Renal and urinary tract surgery

■ Nephrectomy (removal of kidney).

Each type of surgery is carried out by specialist surgeons and their teams, so patients having surgery to the ear, nose and throat will have a different surgical team and operating theatre to patients having surgery on the gastrointestinal system. Nurses who work in theatres may well specialise in the same field as the surgeon and eventually lead a team of nurses who may work only for that surgical specialty.

The nurse caring for a patient undergoing surgery for orthopaedic problems noted above will be expected to have a detailed knowledge of the anatomy and physiology of the musculoskeletal system as well as the surgery involved, including the exact instruments the orthopaedic surgeon might need to carry out the procedure.

In an orthopaedic operating theatre, the noise levels can be quite high due to the tools used, and a study by Siverdeen et al (2008) found that this could lead to potential hearing problems in staff exposed for prolonged periods and that precautions and careful monitoring of noise levels was important.

Safety in the operating theatre

There are a wide range of safety issues in the operating theatre. Given the fact that the environment has highly specialised electrical equipment, anaesthetic gases and has to be infection proof, as a student it is important that you are fully aware of the management of risk in these areas when going either to observe or to experience a full placement.

Your mentor will ensure you are made aware of local policies and procedures with regards to safety in all areas of the operating theatre and its related areas, but we now consider basic information that you can refer to either before or during the placement.

Activity

Review the NMC (2010) Essential Skills Cluster: Infection Prevention and Control.

Once you are aware of the policies, procedures and evidence base for some of the related nursing activities, undertake the following.

Linked to your forthcoming progression point (PP1 and final third year placement for those on the 2004 NMC Standards and Competencies, and PP1, PP2 or final sign off placement for those on the 2010 NMC Standards and Competencies), develop an action plan with your mentor as to the opportunities you will experience while in the operating theatre and how these can be evidenced as a record of your achieving this essential skill cluster. (See Appendix 1 at the end of this chapter for the Infection Prevention and Control Essential Skills Cluster outcomes.)

Infection prevention in the operating theatre

Infection prevention in the operating theatre is achieved through careful use of aseptic techniques in order to prevent contamination of the open wound and isolation of the operative site from the surrounding unsterile physical environment through creating and maintaining a sterile field in which surgery can be performed safely (Weaving et al 2008).

 Activity

Weaving et al's (2008) article is an Open Learning Zone article for qualified nurses but has some excellent learning tasks which you could also undertake. It has a very comprehensive reference list which is an added resource. It can be found in full at:

http://findarticles.com/p/articles/mi_ m0748/is_5_18/ai_n31879368/? tag=content;col1 (accessed December 2011).

Weaving et al (2008:200) talk about a 'back to basics' approach as being 'the key to optimal infection control and prevention in the operating theatre'. They note that the theatre design must first of all make sure that airborne bacteria are removed from the surrounding fields through adequate ventilation throughout the operating theatre suite as a whole (as the theatres connect with each other) as well as it being an environment that is easily cleaned and managed. Good theatre practice is second on their list of important control and prevention activities, being underpinned by a current evidence base and not just custom and practice.

They describe an evidence base regarding preparation of the patient (citing Tanner's (2006) and Tanner et al's (2007) evidence on hair removal and skin preparation) and staff preparation (special clothing and removal of jewellery, hair covering, nail care, etc.). They advocate the wearing of masks, sterile gloves and gowns by staff as a matter of course both for their own protection and that of the patient, underpinned by other evidence. Patient preparation includes the use of special sterile drapes (no touching by non-sterile personnel) and, prior to any management of sterile equipment or field, systematic hand antisepsis (hand scrubbing) with an appropriate solution. This applies to all staff involved in managing the surgical field and the actual surgical procedure. Hand hygiene applies to all personnel in the team. Many hospitals now ensure that even visitors are encouraged to use antiseptic solutions strategically placed throughout the corridors, outside wards and in other areas. Weaving et al (2008:202) also point out that even though surgical instruments arrive sterile, there may still be a risk of contamination and that *'in order to minimise this risk, all members of the operating team need to be proficient in aseptic technique'.*

Activity

Look at the following video clips of handwashing on the ward and the handwash you are expected to undertake in the operating theatre if you are going to assist as a scrub nurse.

A Complete Guide to Hand Washing (University of Leicester): http://www.youtube. com/watch?v=mWe51EKbewk (accessed May 2011).

A Comprehensive Guide to the Surgical Scrub (Whittington Hospital London): http:// www.youtube.com/watch?v=L8OLnyJ3mAc&feature=related (accessed May 2011).

Continued

These are two very good examples of good handwashing practice. Your university may also have its own clinical skills video material – check this out on your virtual learning environment such as BlackBoard.

Under the supervision and direction of your mentor, practice undertaking both types of experiences and discuss what the differences are between normal day-to-day best handwashing practice and that related to the surgical scrub practice of gowning up and putting on sterile gloves for assisting during surgery. What are the challenges you experience in doing a surgical scrub handwash and gowning up/putting on gloves in the theatre environment?

Documentation before, during and after surgery

Accurate and legible record keeping in theatres is very important.

Activity

Before reading this section, review the NMC (2009) Record keeping: guidance for nurses and midwives at:
http://www.nmc-uk.org/Documents/Guidance/nmcGuidanceRecord
KeepingGuidanceforNursesand
Midwives.pdf (accessed May 2011).

Accurate documentation at all stages of the perioperative journey is essential. Healey et al (2008), through a process of change management, updated their perioperative nursing documentation which included an evidence-based approach to perioperative practice, in particular the importance of ensuring a pre- and post-surgery count of all instruments and swabs used during the surgery.

Counting instruments, needles and swabs before surgery begins is critical to the safety of the patient, to ensure that an accurate post-surgical count balances that taken pre-surgery. It is vital that instruments, needles or swabs are not left inside the patient during operations which may involve severe bleeding and the use of many different types of large and small instruments. (See the Association for Perioperative Practice guidelines at Great Ormond Street Hospital: http://www.gosh.nhs.uk/clinical_information/clinical_guidelines/cpg_guideline_00012/#Ref_section (accessed May 2011).)

Activity

Arrange with your mentor to observe the counting and documenting of the instruments and swab both before and after surgery has taken place. If possible, do this both for a very complex surgical intervention and one that is less so.

Many operating theatres have instruments and equipment set aside for teaching purposes. It is good practice if you are in the operating theatre area for the whole of your placement to become familiar with some of these. If you are fortunate to be given an opportunity to scrub up for an operation alongside your mentor, you may also be asked to pass the surgeon specific instruments during the surgery. This may be an agreed final objective for you, and some of you may really like this special environment and wish to work there on qualifying. It is a very rewarding place to work although, as with every specialty, it is not everyone's final employment choice.

Safe positioning of the patient during surgery

Patients arriving in the operating theatre from the anaesthetic room have to placed on an operating theatre table. In order for the surgeon to be able to access the part of the body that is to be operated on, the position the patient is placed in is very important and there are different ones for different types of surgery. It is also important to note that positioning of the patient can have an effect on blood pressure, venous return and ventilation (Hughes & Mardell 2009). Again we can see how important it is that students have the knowledge about normal and disturbed physiology of the body systems as well as anatomy.

When positioning patients on the operating table, it is important that all staff involved adhere to moving and handling regulations and that (Gilmour 2010:23):

the team involved undertake a risk assessment for the moving and handling of each individual patient, and that relevant aids and methods are used to reduce patient movement and potential injury to both staff and patients. An assessment will include the physical condition of the patient, nature of the intervention and individual patient's needs.

If patients are not positioned correctly, it is possible to inflict damage to the patient, such as nerve injuries, due to their relaxed state during surgery. Gilmour (2010:23) states: *'radial nerve injury can occur if the arm is left hanging over the edge of the operating table; ulnar nerve injury due to compression by an inappropriately placed arm support'.*

Common surgical positions are highlighted in Box 8.3. (See Hughes & Mardell (2009) for images of the different positions.)

Box 8.3 Common surgical positions

Supine

Patient is positioned on their back with arms extended on arm boards or alongside their body. This position is used for general abdominal surgery such as a laparotomy, breast surgery or vascular surgery.

Lateral

Patient is placed on their side with additional support for legs (which need to be separated with a pillow), head and all pressure points. This position is used for surgery such as a total hip replacement (arthroplasty) and kidney surgery.

Prone

Patient is placed in the supine position then rolled over onto their front, with head and lower limbs supported with special supports. This position is used for surgery on the spine, neck and buttocks.

Trendelenburg

Patient is positioned as per supine but involves tilting the table head downwards at an angle of 40 degrees. This position is used for abdominal/pelvic/gynaecology procedures. (A reverse of this, where the table is tilted the other way, can also be used but the feet will need to be supported – used for certain head and neck procedures.)

Lithotomy

Patient placed on the table with buttocks at the end of the table and feet placed in fixed stirrups. This position is used for surgery on the perineum, vagina and rectum.

(Adapted from Hughes & Mardell 2009:328–333)

> ✔ **Tip**
>
> During your induction onto the placement, ensure that you make yourself familiar with the moving and handling policy, as well as other teaching and learning packages available for students on the different positioning of patients and the management of risk.

Universal precautions

Universal precautions were introduced in the USA in 1987 initially to manage blood-borne viruses. It was later extended to include all body fluids and matter which could carry pathogenic microorganisms, which in turn could lead to infection. This applied to any environment where this risk was a possibility.

In the operating theatre, it includes hand hygiene and protective clothing such as gloves, masks, eye protection, shoes, hats and gowns. It also covers good sharps practice (needles and syringes) and correct disposal; how to decontaminate equipment; managing used laundry and any clinical waste (such as after an amputation); and spillage of any blood or body fluids/products.

All hospitals are required to have a universal precautions policy, and the Department of Health's (DH) Health and Social Care Act 2008 (DH 2009) came into force in April 2010 for NHS providers and October 2010 for other registered providers: http://www.dh.gov.uk/en/Publicationsandstatistics/Publications/PublicationsPolicyAndGuidance/DH_110288 (accessed May 2011).

An example of the universal precautions and operating theatre practice policy can be seen at this NHS trust document: http://www.ruh.nhs.uk/about/policies/documents/clinical_policies/local/416_Theatre_Practice_Policy.pdf (accessed May 2011).

> 🖎 **Activity**
>
> It is essential that you discuss the universal precautions policy for your placement in the perioperative environment. Ensure that it becomes one of your learning goals, as infection prevention and control is one of the key areas of the essential skills clusters outcomes that you have to become competent in (see Box 8.3).
>
> Read the articles by Cutter and Jordan (2004) and Gammon et al (2007) (see References) which illustrate research studies undertaken to examine compliance with standard/universal infection control policies.

Discharge of the patient from the operating theatre

Following completion of surgery, the anaesthetist will already be starting the process of lightening the anaesthesia given to the patient, who will be transferred from the operating theatre (following the counting of the instruments and swabs), ensuring the safety of the patient and any equipment attached such as intravenous fluids, catheters and drains, into the recovery area or ward where there may be other patients also in the recovery stage. This is the next part of the patient journey, discussed in Chapter 9.

Summary

This chapter has given you an insight into what you can learn in the operating theatre, either as part of your surgical ward experience or on a full placement.

References

Audit Commission 2001 Day Surgery; Review of National Findings, Audit Commission, London.

Cutter, J., Jordan, S., 2004. Uptake of guidelines to avoid and report exposure to blood and body fluids. Journal of Advanced Nursing 46 (4), 441–452.

Department of Health, 2009. The Health and Social Care Act 2008: code of practice for health and adult social care on the prevention and control of infections and related guidance. DH, London.

Gammon, J., Morgan-Samuel, H., Gould, D., 2007. A review of the evidence for suboptimal compliance of healthcare practitioners to standard/universal infection control precautions. Journal of Clinical Nursing 17, 157–167.

Gilmour, D., 2010. Perioperative care. In: Pudner, R. (Ed.), Nursing the surgical patient, 3rd ed. Baillière Tindall, Edinburgh.

Healey, K., Hegarty, J., Keating, G., et al., 2008. The change experience: how we updated our perioperative nursing documentation. Journal of Perioperative Practice 18 (4), 163–166.

Hughes, S.J., Mardell, A., 2009. Oxford handbook of perioperative practice. Oxford University Press, Oxford.

Mitchell, L., Finn, R., 2008. Non-technical skills of the operating theatre scrub nurses: literature review. Journal of Advanced Nursing 63 (1), 15–24.

Mitchell, M., 2010. A patient-centred approach to day surgery nursing. Nursing Standard 24 (44), 40–46.

Mottram, A., 2011. Like a trip to McDonald's: a grounded theory study of patient experiences of day surgery. International Journal of Nursing Studies 48 (2), 165–174.

Nursing and Midwifery Council, 2009. Record keeping: guidance for nurses and midwives. NMC, London.

Nursing and Midwifery Council, 2010. Standards for pre-registration nursing education. NMC, London.

Oakley, M., 2010. Day surgery. In: Pudner, R. (Ed.), Nursing the surgical patient, 3rd ed. Baillière Tindall, Edinburgh.

Siverdeen, Z., Ali, A., Lakdawala, A.S., McKay, C., 2008. Exposure to noise in orthopaedic theatres – do we need protection? International Journal of Clinical Practice 62 (11), 1720–1722.

Tanner, J., 2006. Surgical gloves: perforation and protection. Journal of Perioperative Practice 16 (1), 148–152.

Tanner, J., Moncaster, K., Woodings, D., 2007. Perioperative hair removal: a systematic review. Journal of Perioperative Practice 17 (3), 118–132.

Weaving, P., Cox, F., Milton, S., 2008. Infection prevention and control in the operating theatre: reducing the risk of surgical site infections (SSIs). Journal of Perioperative Practice 18 (5), 199–204.

Further reading

Hughes, S., 2006. Evaluating operating theatre experience. Journal of Perioperative Practice 16 (6), 290–298.

Hughes, S., Mardell, A., 2009. Oxford handbook of perioperative practice. Oxford University Press, Oxford.

Sampson, H., 2006. Introducing student nurses to operating department nursing. Journal of Perioperative Practice 16 (2), 87–94.

Wicker, P., O'Neill, J., 2010. Caring for the perioperative patient, 2nd ed. Wiley-Blackwell, Oxford.

Websites

World Health Organisation – 10 facts on surgical safety: http://www.who.int/features/factfiles/safe_surgery/en/ (accessed December 2011).

Association for Perioperative Practitioners information: http://www.afpp.org.uk/about-AfPP (accessed December 2011).

The surgical count (instruments and swabs): http://www.gosh.nhs.uk/clinical_information/clinical_guidelines/cpg_guideline_00012 (accessed December 2011).

Royal College of Physicians UK latex allergy information and guidance: http://www.rcplondon.ac.uk/resources/latex-allergy-guideline (accessed May 2011).

Resuscitation Council UK guidelines on anaphylaxis: http://www.resus.org.uk/pages/reaction.pdf (accessed December 2011).

World Health Organisation safety checklist for operating theatre practice and implementation manual: http://www.who.int/patientsafety/safesurgery/tools_resources/SSSL_Checklist_finalJun08.pdf and http://www.who.int/patientsafety/safesurgery/tools_resources/SSSL_Manual_finalJun08.pdf (accessed December 2011).

For details about this and a wide range of other excellent perioperative care resources, access the CETL website at City University London: http://www.cetl.org.uk/learning/tutorials.html and the linked online resource: http://www.cetl.org.uk/learning/perioperative-care/player.html (accessed May 2011). This site has information sheets and video/audio material on all stages of the perioperative care journey as well as quizzes and tests to check your learning.

http://www.who.int/features/factfiles/safe_surgery/en/ (accessed December 2011).

http://www.youtube.com/watch?v=U6p5LEG04mU&feature=related (accessed December 2011).

http://www.youtube.com/watch?v=CsNpfMldtyk (accessed December 2011).

Appendix 1

Specific learning experiences in the operating theatre: checklist of possible learning outcomes

■ To become familiar with the layout of the operating theatre and where everything is kept, such as equipment and various intravenous fluids.

■ To gain experience working in a multidisciplinary team and understand the role of the theatre team as well as other health professionals who have close links to patient care in the theatre, such as radiographers or pathologists.

■ To gain an understanding of the importance of infection prevention and control as well as universal precautions and the sterilisation of equipment and surgical packs.

■ To gain an understanding of the importance of maintaining accurate documentation and recording of events in the operating theatre.

■ To gain experience of effective communication to ensure patient safety and to be a patient advocate at all times.

■ To gain experience in managing the holistic care of the patient during surgery, maintaining their dignity and also demonstrating an awareness of any special cultural needs and/or special needs such as patients with learning difficulties, loss of hearing, vision or speech.

Appendix 1—cont'd

- To demonstrate understanding and practice of asepsis and aseptic technique.
- To observe and/or perform surgical scrub and putting on gown and gloves.
- To gain an understanding of and demonstrate implementation of all correct procedures with regards to the surgical field, including instruments, needles and swabs, types of sutures and drains used.
- To demonstrate a knowledge of the various positions that patients are placed in on the operating table and the reasons why as well as for what surgical procedures.

9 Recovery from surgery

Introduction

A patient's recovery from surgery begins as soon as the actual surgical procedure is completed and the patient leaves the operating theatre. At this stage, the anaesthetist along with the team of nurses and other healthcare practitioners will be responsible for managing the immediate postoperative recovery of the patient. Once the anaesthetist in charge is satisfied that the patient has overcome the immediate effects of the surgery, he/she will decide whether the patient can be transferred safely back to their original ward.

In some cases, due to postoperative needs, the patient may be transferred to a high-dependency unit or intensive care unit. Under some circumstances, such as major chest surgery or prolonged anaesthesia, this will have been predicted and staff in those units will already be prepared to receive the patient.

This chapter focuses on two areas for postoperative recovery: the recovery room in the immediate postoperative period and recovery on the ward for the rest of the postoperative period until discharged home from hospital. Allvin et al (2006) cite studies about ambulatory (day care) surgery where these two areas are added to by a third one (what they call the late phase of postoperative recovery); 'from discharge until the patients reach preoperative health and well-being' (2006:553). We discuss this more fully in Chapter 10.

Care of the patient in the recovery room: immediately postoperative

The postoperative stage of patient care begins as soon as the patient is transferred from the theatre to the recovery area/room. These are normally purpose-built rooms set up with the right equipment and resources and staffed by experienced recovery room nurses. Gilmour (2010) cites the view of the Association of Anaesthetists of Great Britain and Ireland (AAGBI) *'that patients must be observed on a one to one nurse:patient ratio until the patient has regained airway control, is cardiovascularly stable and can communicate'* (AAGBI 2002).

We can therefore identify that the nurse must focus on three areas of physiological monitoring in the immediate postoperative transfer period, namely airway, breathing and circulation. The handover from the theatre nurse/anaesthetist also includes detailed information about the patient, their surgery, their vital signs, any medication already given, any IVs in progress, any catheters or drains and any special instructions regarding their immediate monitoring and management (Gilmour 2010).

Depending on when you undertake this placement, most of you will have been taught some clinical skills in a safe environment such as a clinical skills laboratory at university. The main skills will initially be recording of temperature, pulse and respiration as well as blood pressure. These become vital skills in the immediate postoperative period, both manually and electronically where many patients are recorded by special monitors and equipment which you can observe.

Observations in the immediate postoperative period

Amos and Waugh (2007) refer to the priorities of the immediate postoperative recovery as defined by the Scottish Intercollegiate Guidelines Network (2004) as airway, breathing and circulation (see http://www.sign.ac.uk/pdf/sign77.pdf (accessed May 2011)).

Airway

The patient's airway must be kept clear at all times, and initially they may have an airway (Guedal) in place (in situ) to help keep the airway patent and to enable adequate ventilation and breathing.

It is important to ensure that the patient's position is not hampering the airway and, unless contraindicated such as in a total hip replacement where rolling onto their side is not an option, the patient can be nursed in the recovery position – on their side or supine, depending on instructions from the surgical team.

Oxygen is given immediately either with a mask or nasal cannulae, *'normally at 40%. Contraindications include chronic obstructive airways disease or when a prescribed percentage of oxygen is required. A pulse oximeter is attached to monitor oxygen levels'* (Gilmour 2010:28).

⬗ Activity

Discuss with your mentor your responsibilities in the immediate care of patients in the recovery room. This is an ideal opportunity to develop not only your clinical skills but also your communication skills in a different environment. Patients are very vulnerable at this time and many will wake up worried about what has happened during surgery. Make sure you focus on learning how to communicate with patients using various senses and also communicate any concerns the patient may experience with your mentor or a qualified member of the recovery team.

Read an up-to-date evidence-based book on clinical skills and postoperative care of the patient and aim to make maximum use of materials for students in the learning environment (see Further Reading list).

Breathing

It is important to check that the patient's breathing is even and not noisy, which could indicate a possible obstruction, but take into account that 'complete obstruction is characterised by silence' (Gilmour 2010:29). It is important to check the skin colour, especially the lips and nail beds, which may indicate cyanosis. (Link this back to preoperative preparation where make up and nail varnish have to be removed – see Ch. 6.)

As well as checking for any airway/breathing obstruction and slow breathing, breathing may also become rapid and the patient might be gasping for breath. Any sudden change you observe must be reported immediately to the qualified nurse responsible for the patient and/or the anaesthetist in order that immediate remedial action can take place.

Circulation

Monitoring of the pulse and blood pressure is an essential observation and some patients will have electronic monitoring of their observations to aid you in maintaining patient safety postoperatively.

As the patient is likely to have wounds and drains, it is important that these are also checked as per instructions, obviously not disturbing any wound dressings while doing so. A dressing saturated with blood requiring additional dressings and packing is an indication that the patient may be haemorrhaging – this will be accompanied by a raised rapid pulse rate and a sudden drop in blood pressure.

If a patient has had a below-the-knee amputation, for example, the surface of the dressing may seem as if there is no increased blood loss despite physical signs of raised rapid pulse rate and dropping blood pressure. If the patient is supine, it is important to also check beneath the leg as blood may be pooling underneath, soaking the sheets rather than the dressing. This is an example from our own experience in nursing practice, with the result that the patient had to be immediately taken back to the operating theatre as a blood vessel required diathermy.

The anaesthetist will have written in the patient's notes the exact postoperative care required with regards to observations and medications, and the medication (prescription) sheet will detail specific postoperative analgesia. Managing a patient's pain is a major aspect of postoperative care, as pain can not only cause the patient some distress but also impact on postoperative physiological responses.

Pain management in the immediate recovery period

Pain is an unavoidable side effect following surgery, but how people cope with this will differ according to gender, age, psychological and cultural factors together with individual coping mechanism (Hughes 2004). The management of pain will already have been discussed with the patient preoperatively unless, of course, the patient was admitted as an emergency, when pain relief will already have commenced.

In the immediate postoperative period in the recovery room, the patient may not easily be able to articulate their pain levels, due to being drowsy or a fear of moving. Other non-verbal cues may be indicative of the need for pain relief, such as restlessness. A study by Heikkinen et al (2005) found that assessment of pain for prostatectomy patients in the recovery room was possible using pain assessment tools even though the patient may be sedated, but that there was inconclusive evidence as to which was best. They maintained that the key issue was 'the pain is assessed systematically and that both nurse and patient understand the meaning of the assessment' (2005:598).

Activity

Discuss with your mentor whether they use a pain assessment tool in the recovery room and, if yes, agree to use this with a patient under supervision. If a pain tool is not used, discuss why not and how the nurses know if a patient is in pain.

You may choose to consider evaluating pain assessment and management in the immediate postoperative period as a topic for an evidence-based practice assignment or as a presentation to your peers.

Analgesia can be administered via a number of different routes and techniques (Gilmour 2010, Amos & Waugh 2007). These are:

- *intramuscular injection*
- *intravenous bolus*
- *intravenous patient-controlled analgesia (PCA)*
- *epidural*
- *rectally*
- *orally*
- *subcutaneously.*

When caring for a patient either pre- or postoperatively, it is important that you familiarise yourself with all of these in order to ensure effective communication and discussion with the patient as well as ensuring evidence-based nursing care delivery. Knowing how each of these work in controlling pain should also be supported by knowing the physiological effects.

If the surgery is major, it is likely that the route of administration will be the intravenous PCA, given that this avoids use of injections and, importantly, the patient feels in control of their own pain management. The effectiveness of any pain management should be evident when the patient can move more easily and not be afraid to move, as well as being less anxious. In addition, there may be a change in the patient's observations, for example the pulse rate might have been raised and rapid before being given pain relief due to the effect of the pain stressor on the body, and this will stabilise.

Regardless of the extent of the surgical intervention, the patient will experience some degree of pain. It is important at this stage to remember that some patients may not be able to articulate that they are in pain and that physiological signs and symptoms will be the first identification. Continual observation and reassurance by the nurse is essential to the patient's wellbeing. We return to this topic again when the patient has been returned to the ward area.

Managing postoperative nausea and vomiting (PONV)

Following surgery, this remains a common complication (Gibson 2006) and is very distressing for the patient. It may add to any postoperative pain they have due to the 'retching' movements during vomiting and the heart rate and blood pressure may be increased (DeLeskey 2009). Anaesthetics used during surgery contribute to this postoperative problem but it can also be a side effect of strong analgesics used postoperatively such as those with an opioid base.

 Activity

Read about the physiology of pain and make notes about the impact of surgery on the body's normal response to pain.

Determine which route for analgesia would be appropriate for a range of surgical situations.

Read Allen D (2005:133–148) (see References) to help you with this activity.

Monitoring the patient for other potential immediate postoperative complications

Two other main potential complications can occur in the immediate recovery period: hypothermia and wound haemorrhage (see above for one possible example affecting the circulatory system).

Wicker and Cox (2010:390) identify three possible causes of hypothermia postoperatively, namely *'vasodilation or vasoconstriction, a recognised complication following surgery and a large infusion of blood and fluids'*. Postoperatively, the patient must be kept warm and they advise that a 'space blanket' should be applied and that *'the room environment should be kept at a warm temperature, above 21 degrees C'* (2010:387). However, patients must not be heated up too quickly either.

Wound haemorrhage can occur in the immediate postoperative recovery period

through *'inadequate wound closure, leaking vascular anastomosis and inadequate homeostasis'* (Wicker & Cox 2010:390) and you need to be careful to observe any wounds for signs of these. Inform your mentor immediately if you notice any signs of haemorrhage at the wound site or other indications (as discussed above) for tachycardia and hypotension.

Patients must be physiologically stable before they leave the recovery room and they must be awake and have normal airway reflexes (Wicker & Cox 2010) (see Box 9.1).

Discharge from the post-operative recovery room

The length of time spent in this area will depend on issues such as type of anaesthesia, type of surgery, length of surgery and the postoperative recovery of the patient. The anaesthetist will make that

---

Box 9.1 Discharge from post-anaesthetic recovery

- *The patient is fully conscious and can respond to voice or light touch, is able to maintain a clear airway and has a normal cough reflex.*
- *Respiration and oxygen saturation are satisfactory (10–20 breaths per minute and SpO_2 is >92%).*
- *The cardiovascular system is stable with no unexplained cardiac irregularity or persistent bleeding. The patient's pulse and blood pressure should approximate to normal preoperative values or should be at a value commensurate with the planned postoperative care.*
- *Pain and emesis should be controlled and suitable analgesic and antiemetic regimens prescribed*
- *Temperature should be within acceptable limits (>36°C).*
- *Oxygen and fluid therapy should be prescribed as required.*

Prior to discharge, the recovery staff should record in the notes that patients have met these criteria. If a patient does not meet these criteria, they should be assessed by the anaesthetist responsible either for the procedure or post-anaesthetic recovery with a view to upgrade to level 2 or 3 care (see full document for further details).

(From Scottish Intercollegiate Guidelines Network 2002:3)

decision based on the recovery nurse's assessment and observations (Smith & Hardy 2007). The ward nurse will receive the handover of the patient from the recovery nurse with a complete report of the surgery, the postoperative care instructions, the current condition of the patient and any medication he/she has been given. Explanations of what is going on will be given to the patient at this time, and many patients will recognise the nurse who has come for them from the ward, especially if it is their named nurse. This is an ideal opportunity for you to undertake a patient transfer back to the ward with your mentor or another member of the ward team.

> ### ✔ Tip
>
> For details about this and a wide range of other excellent perioperative care resources, access the CETL website at City University London:
> http://www.cetl.org.uk/learning/tutorials.html (accessed May 2011).
>
> and this linked online resource:
> http://www.cetl.org.uk/learning/perioperative-care/player.html (accessed May 2011).
>
> This site has information sheets and video/audio material on all stages of the perioperative care journey and quizzes and tests to check out your learning.

Care of the patient postoperatively: back on the ward

Once a patient has left the ward for the operating theatre, the bed area is prepared for their return. If the patient's bed has been taken to the recovery room, then he/she will be returning on that bed. The nurse collecting the patient from theatre must take with them a vomit bowl, a pair of gloves (universal precautions), a Guedel airway and a hand-held ventilation Ambu bag (or similar).

Preparation of the bed area in the ward includes checking the oxygen supply (and making sure there is an oxygen mask and proper tubing); checking the suction system/machine and its proper tubing; making sure there is equipment to take blood pressure; and, if necessary, a pulse oximeter to measure oxygen saturation levels. An IV stand may be required if a patient has undergone major surgery as they are most likely to return from the operating theatre with intravenous fluids.

On return to the ward, the nurse takes immediate postoperative observations. Charts are used to record details of temperature, pulse and respiration, fluid balance and, depending on the nature of the surgery, other charts as appropriate.

In patients who have been admitted for day care surgery, the same observations are undertaken on the patient's return, but there will usually not be intravenous fluids to consider as patients having this kind of surgery don't require them.

All observations are recorded on the charts and in the nursing care documentation.

General principles of care in the first 24 hours postoperatively

According to Endacott et al (2009), there are key care steps in the first 24 hours postoperatively and these can be used to help focus on the priorities for the ward nurse on the patient's return from theatre. We return to these in Section 3 where we introduce you to three patients and their perioperative journeys along with learning opportunities that you can pursue in their care.

Steps for postoperative care in the first 24 hours (adapted from Endacott et al 2009)

Step 1: safe transfer and communication

This involves safe transfer of the patient from the recovery room staff to ward staff and return to the ward. Essential information has to be handed over at this time (see above). This is important in order to ensure there is effective communication between care areas but it is also important for patients to know they are going back to the ward and that the surgery is very much over.

Step 2: vital signs and consciousness

Before leaving the operating theatre, all vital signs related to airway, breathing and circulation will have been checked, and these are also checked during transfer and on immediate return to the ward. Consciousness levels are checked as well.

Step 3: early warning score systems

Many of these observations are also included in the early warning score systems (Johnstone et al 2007) which are designed as triggers to indicate a deterioration in a patient's condition. Johnstone et al (2007:221) state that:

> As a result of the reduction in the number of acute beds within the NHS trusts, medical and surgical wards are now tending to have a higher number of sicker and more dependent patients … These patients are at greater risk of having a period of critical illness within these general wards and there is a growing recognition that several indicators of acute deterioration are being missed by nurses and doctors.

There are short courses and longer modules that give training in use of these early warning score systems, and Preston and Flynn (2010) identified some key points in their review of the evidence of the effectiveness and use of these tools (see Box 9.2).

Box 9.2 Review of the evidence: observations in acute care – an evidence-based approach to patient safety

1. *Doing observations in acute care is crucial for detecting early signs of deterioration.*
2. *Nurses need a sound knowledge of physiological compensatory mechanisms to facilitate accurate detection of changes in temperature, pulse and respiration, blood pressure, blood glucose levels, neurological function and blood oxygen saturation levels.*
3. *Recording the respiratory rate is a sensitive indicator of clinical deterioration.*
4. *Early warning systems, including the Glasgow Coma Scale, are tools to aid identification of patients at risk of adverse clinical situations (cardiac arrest, raised intracranial pressure, sepsis).*
5. *ALERT (Acute Life-threatening Events – Recognition and Treatment) courses and simulation exercises conducted in a safe environment and development of critical thinking skills that underpin appropriate recognition and reporting of clinical deterioration.*
6. *Observations should be assessed by a qualified nurse if detection of patient deterioration is to be consistent in acute care.*

(From Preston & Flynn (2010:442–447))

Activity

Determine how many different tools are available in your placement which give an indication of a change in the postoperative status of patients in that area.

Set a learning goal during your placement that you will observe the use of the main early warning score system, and make a contribution to assessing the status of a patient by completing this under the supervision of your mentor.

Step 4: other observations Endacott et al (2009) recommend checking pulse rate and blood pressure every 15 minutes for the first hour, then every 30 minutes for 2 hours. After that, the observation rate can be increased or reduced according to the patient's condition. At the same time, the skin should be observed for paleness, sweating and peripheral vasoconstriction (cold extremities). Patients who have had surgery will have surgical incisions (wounds) that will need to be observed for blood loss, and sometimes they will leave the recovery room with their external dressing marked for where the blood had been oozing through (this is undertaken carefully so as not to harm the patient). This line around the 'blood mark' can then be watched for any increase in size over the first 24 hours. Many surgical procedures, however, do not have large wounds so there is minimal dressing applied and minimal bleeding.

Step 5: major complications One of the major complications to occur postoperatively is postoperative shock. Gibson (2006:921) makes the following observation with regards to this and its cause:

> When the patient returns from theatre to the ward, they require frequent observations for signs of impending

shock or haemorrhage. As blood pressure continues to rise, there is a continued risk of reactionary haemorrhage for the first 24 hours. Hypovolaemic shock may also occur due to a slow, continuous loss of fluid; this might be a slowly bleeding vessel or the pooling of fluid in the gastrointestinal tract during the paralytic ileus that occurs as a consequence of surgery. The loss of fluid may be detected as soakage on the dressing or blood in the wound drains, but if the patient is bleeding into a body cavity or losing fluid into the gut it may be less obvious. Distinction should also be made between hypovolaemic shock and other forms of shock, i.e. cardiogenic, septic, anaphylactic and neurogenic.

Undertaking nursing observations as prescribed in this first 24-hour period is therefore vital to detect shock and haemorrhage (see Gibson & Magowan 2011).

 Activity

Find out what cardiogenic, septic, anaphylactic and neurogenic shock are. Further discussion on these is found later in this book and in the case studies in Section 3.

Patients returning after major surgery may be prescribed intravenous fluids, and sometimes a blood transfusion may be in progress. If the latter, then it is essential to undertake appropriate observations to ensure any adverse reactions to the blood are noted. Transfusion reactions can vary from a mild to a severe life-threatening situation. Symptoms range from a mild fever and pruritus to rigors, tachycardia and respiratory distress – shortness of breath due to anaphylaxis (Oldham et al 2009).

Find out the potential problems associated with a blood transfusion and visit the hospital blood bank to find out the correct procedure for checking out blood for patients. Discuss the procedure with your mentor and ask if you can participate in this activity.

The articles by Gray et al (2008) and Oldham et al (2009) will help you understand the evidence base to changes in blood transfusion practice.

The tutorial on this CETL website is an excellent resource as well:

http://www.cetl.org.uk/learning/blood-transfusion/player.html (accessed December 2011).

Fluid intake and output are also monitored. For many patients, it is difficult to pass urine in the immediate stage postoperatively, not least because many are frightened to move if they have a wound which causes them pain on movement. For some, this problem does not last very long and they will manage to pass urine. If they still haven't passed urine 4–6 hours postoperatively (but their observations regarding circulation and breathing have been satisfactory during this time), this must be reported to the medical staff. If patients have a catheter in situ then it is easier to see if they are passing urine and, most importantly, how much per hour. If the output is less than 4 ml/kg of body weight per hour, this also needs to be reported. It is essential that the function of the kidneys is maintained postoperatively.

Drainage from any wound also needs to be observed as does any fluid loss from a nasogastric tube. If excessive, this needs to be reported as well.

Step 6: pain Levels of postoperative pain depend on the nature of the surgery and, of course, the individual patient. Whatever the

type of surgery, pain levels need to be assessed and recorded and medication given. Pain assessment tools can be useful such as the 'faces' scale or a numerical one to rate the level of pain between 0 and 10 where $0 =$ no pain and $10 =$ worst pain imaginable (Bell & Duffy 2009).

For patients who have had major surgery, a PCA system may be prescribed and inserted in the operating theatre/recovery room and the patient may already have been made aware of having this in the preoperative phase.

Bell and Duffy (2009:156), however, in their review on the issue of pain assessment and management in surgical nursing found that '*despite all the research carried out on pain assessment and management, very little has changed in practice*'. They conclude that there appears to be two significant barriers to effective practice (although cautioned that it was a multidisciplinary issue to solve), namely '*the beliefs and attitudes of both patients and nurses towards pain management and nurses' time management*'.

⟩ **Activity**

Read Bell and Duffy (2009) (see References) and decide if this is a good literature review or not and whether your experience in a surgical placement of any kind can be related to their findings. Discuss with your mentor and share with others in the placement your evidence base for pain assessment and management. This is a valuable topic to explore as pain management extends beyond the boundaries of surgery and the principles of care can be applied to other contexts.

If a patient has a PCA in place, this will have been explained to them preoperatively and they will have been shown the machine.

Obviously, if a patient was admitted as an emergency, this would not have been an immediate priority, so a careful explanation of what it is and how to use it will have to be completed by the nurse responsible for the patient's care both in the recovery and ward areas.

Observations of the patient using the PCA will include observing for any adverse effects such as increased sedation, respiratory depression, nausea, pruritus, urine retention and hallucinations/confusion (NHS Quality Improvement Scotland 2004).

The types of medication used postoperatively will depend on the nature of the surgery and immediate postoperative care needs, and will change as a patient progresses postoperatively. The main ones in the immediate postoperative period, if the surgery warrants it, are opioids and antiemetics. Opioids are given intravenously in the recovery room. See Box 9.3 for a description of the rationale and additional information about opioids and the use of a PCA.

There is a large body of literature available on pain management and control both from nursing and medical professionals. Some helpful resources can be found in the Further Reading section.

Further information is also considered below in the section on care after 24 hours.

Step 7: medication In the immediate postoperative recovery period, it is important to ensure that patients are given the medication they normally take in order to avoid possible side effects from withdrawal. For example, if a patient takes insulin for long-standing diabetes, preoperative and postoperative precautions will be taken. But what happens to the patient's normal medication regimen during surgery if they are unable to eat or drink? In the case of insulin, the patient does not have to be able to eat or drink in order to receive the drug. However, with insulin-dependent diabetes, there are additional and potentially life-threatening issues to take into consideration. The patient's specific needs will be assessed preoperatively and information gained on whether the diabetes is controlled by diet, tablets (hypoglycaemic) or insulin. It may be that a combination of these is being used. It is also important for the anaesthetist to find out whether the patient is suffering from any of the complications of diabetes, such as hypertension, peripheral vascular disease or renal problems, all of which

---

Box 9.3 Providing analgesia: use of IV opioids postoperatively

'This is the ideal route because onset of action is rapid (less than 10 minutes) which is an advantage for patients in acute pain (Scott 2009) .... The IV route of administration is preferred as absorption of an IM [intramuscular] dose may be erratic because of poor blood supply in a recovering postoperative patient. IV opioid patient-controlled analgesia (PCA) is popular in recovery since it allows the patients to titrate small doses of analgesia themselves, according to the pain they feel, giving an accurate level of analgesia. Before commencing PCA, patients require a loading dose of opioid to ensure that pain is controlled with minimal side effects (Chumbley 2009) .... Patients should be educated preoperatively so that they are aware that only they must press the bolus request button, that addiction and overdose are very rare and that the device will make a noise when they request a dose – it is not an alarm to indicate malfunction.'

(From Wicker & Cox 2010:400)

influence the choice of anaesthetic and mode of anaesthesia. Generally, most patients who have diabetes are scheduled to be first on the operating list whenever possible and medication is continued as far as possible on the day of surgery. Following admission to hospital, the patient's sugar level will be monitored closely. See the CETL website for information on how to monitor blood glucose levels: http://www.cetl.org.uk/learning/blood-glucose-monitoring/player.html (accessed June 2011).

📎 Activity

Find out from the literature, ward protocols and other information what the pre- and postoperative requirements are for a patient who has diabetes and is insulin dependent.

Identify key areas of pre- and postoperative care and devise a care plan for a patient going for surgery who cannot eat or drink for at least 24 hours postoperatively and 6 hours preoperatively. The information in Box 9.4 will help you with this care plan.

Access the CETL website for more information on blood glucose monitoring:

http://www.cetl.org.uk/learning/blood-glucose-monitoring/player.html (accessed December 2011).

Box 9.4 Diabetes, insulin and perioperative care

General measures for diabetic patients

- Regularly monitor blood sugar until the patient's routine is back to normal – eating and drinking normally and taking their usual insulin or oral hypoglycaemic agents. Frequency of blood glucose measurement will depend on the exact situation and trends exhibited by the patient but generally should be done 1–2 hourly preoperatively with increased frequency if the situation is not stable.

- Do not discharge any patient home unless certain that the blood sugar is controlled and the patient is able to manage their diabetes.

- Hypoglycaemia is an important and life-threatening complication. It may be defined as blood sugar less than 4 mmol/L. It is usually caused by an imbalance of too little food versus too much insulin or oral hypoglycaemia. It may present with sweating, tachycardia, agitation or confusion, fits or unconsciousness. Many diabetic patients will recognise impending hypoglycaemia and will take action to avoid it. If able to eat and drink, give a glass of Lucozade or juice (non-diet) followed by a sandwich or toast. If glucose is less that 2, or the patient is confused, difficult to rouse or unconscious then call immediate medical help. Give 20–50 ml of 50% dextrose IV (repeated if necessary). If the patient is unconscious, attend to the basics of airway, breathing and circulation. If IV access is not available, give glucagon 1 mg intramuscularly.

Continued

Box 9.4 Diabetes, insulin and perioperative care—cont'd

■ Any diabetic patient undergoing prolonged fasting (more than one missed meal) requires glucose–potassium–insulin (GKI) or sliding scale management. GKI has been shown to provide better glycaemic control than the sliding scale.

Important note: It is not the responsibility of the student nurse to give the medication specified in this extracted guidance – but you may observe the practice and certainly be able to recognise when a diabetic patient requires professional help. It is important to note that the information here is for general care of any diabetic patient and not for the postoperative period when additional care is required, especially for those taking insulin. The sliding scale refers to the giving of insulin and/or dextrose and potassium separately on a sliding scale of dosage depending on blood glucose levels.

(Adapted from NHS Forth Valley 2009)

Step 8: maintaining observations It is important to maintain observations as per postoperative instructions, the nature of the surgery and progress of the patient. An increase in pulse and lowering of blood pressure might be caused by blood loss or haemorrhage, possibly due to a blood vessel not being 'tied off' or ligated during surgery. This requires a return to the operating theatre. Other indications of excess bleeding could be restlessness and cold and clammy skin in addition to the changes in pulse and blood pressure.

Temperature observation is important in the immediate postoperative period, especially for patients who have had major thoracic or abdominal surgery, due to 'prolonged surgery and exposure of thoracic or abdominal contents resulting in significant loss of body heat' (Torrance & Serginson 1999:58).

Observation of respiration rate could show early indication of hypoxia or lack of oxygen, requiring an increase in oxygen given or commencement of oxygen therapy via nasal cannulae or face masks. It is important, however, to note that this is not possible for patients who have chronic obstructive airways disease (COAD) because such patients are used to 'a low concentration of oxygen for their respiratory drive and in such cases an oxygen concentration that is too high can depress ventilation' (Torrance & Surginson 1999:58).

Activity

It can be seen from this brief insight into postoperative observations the importance of understanding normal physiology in order to understand what happens when changes occur.

Ensure that you read your notes on the normal physiology of body systems prior to your clinical placement and work out what happens if, for example, there is severe and sudden blood loss, or a patient develops a high temperature. Examples of books to read can be found in the Further Reading list. Read the experience of a student nurse whilst on clinical placement and what he learnt about the importance of observations: http://nursingstandard.rcnpublishing.co.uk/students/clinical-placements/professional-development/clinical-learning-curves/appearances-can-be-deceptive-with-a-post-operative-patient (Accessed June 2011)

Step 9: infection control and prevention practices Preventing infection is one of the most important postoperative care activities, and as such all personnel involved in patient care need to adopt effective and protocol-driven handwashing practices as a normal day-to-day activity rather than just as part of an aseptic technique (see Ch. 8 for handwashing practice in the operating theatre).

Bennallick and King (2009:47) state that *'infection prevention and control can be defined as a series of strategies and practices that aim to reduce the risk of infection to staff, patients and others where care is delivered'*. They point out a number of essential skills that they believe help prevent the transmission of organisms which are associated with healthcare-associated infections, namely (2009:47):

- *handwashing*
- *putting on sterile and non-sterile gloves*
- *use of disposable aprons*
- *use and disposal of sharps*
- *waste disposal*
- *dealing with spillages*
- *providing source isolation*
- *aseptic technique.*

Activity

Access this report and consider the implications for organisations such as hospitals and the perioperative environments.

http://www.dh.gov.uk/en/
Publicationsandstatistics/
Publications/PublicationsPolicy
AndGuidance/DH_122604 (accessed June 2011).

The consequences of healthcare-associated infection are discussed in this learning resource from CETL:

http://www.cetl.org.uk/learning/
healthcare_associated_infections/
player.html (accessed June 2011).

The Department of Health (DH 2010) introduced a new code of practice in 2010 on the prevention and control of infections in health and social care that was implemented on 1 April 2011. Many hospitals had already adopted principles of good practice in the use of antibacterial handwashing gels, with stations placed strategically to ensure that not only staff use these gels but also the general public visiting the hospital environment. Antibacterial handwashing

Activity

Make a plan to learn how to develop your competence in each of the areas in the bullet list above. A good clinical skills nursing book can help you with the steps involved, as can the simulated learning environment of the clinical skills laboratory.

Check out the following CETL links for helpful information on some of these practices:

Use and disposal of sharps: http://www.
cetl.org.uk/learning/sharps-disposal/
player.html (accessed June 2011).

Aseptic technique (also includes disposal of waste and putting on sterile gloves): http://www.cetl.org.uk/
learning/aseptic-dressing-technique/
player.html (accessed June 2011).

If you have already had experience in the operating theatre, you will have gained skills in putting on gloves, disposing of sharps, dealing with spillages and waste disposal, as well as practising a very specific technique for handwashing. The websites above are excellent resources for learning and testing knowledge on a range of topics connected to a surgical nursing placement as well as other placements you may be allocated to during the course of your study.

gels can also be bought in supermarkets and many people now carry them as part of normal day-to-day practice.

Step 10: essential care in the immediate postoperative period It is important to ensure that all essential personal care is given postoperatively, but ensuring that specific postoperative instructions relevant to the surgical intervention are not compromised in the process.

One of the problems for patients postoperatively is a dry mouth, caused by not drinking and/or perioperative medication which causes lack of saliva. Maintaining good oral hygiene is essential for the wellbeing of patients until they are able to do this for themselves. If a patient has dentures and is fully conscious, ensure they are cleaned before inserting into the mouth and, if nauseated, the patient may choose to wait until they feel better before wanting them in. Sometimes it helps to have their dentures in so they can speak clearly and be understood. If in doubt about inserting them during the first 24 hours postoperatively, check with a qualified member of staff. The articles by Huskinson and Lloyd (2009) and the Royal College of Nursing (RCN) (Heath et al 2011) (see References) discuss the importance of oral health for patients.

Depending on the severity and nature of the surgery, patients may wish to have their own night clothes to replace their surgical gowns. A wash of the hands and face is also welcomed by many patients if they are fully conscious, making them feel refreshed and 'normal' again.

Care of the patient after the first 24 hours postoperatively

The majority of steps highlighted above will continue in one form or another until the patient's discharge home from hospital. We can, however, focus on key postoperative care issues in this section that will help you to care for a patient who has undergone surgery. It is not possible to focus on specific types of surgery here, but we consider broad areas in Section 3 where the principles of practice are considered in more specific contexts and for different types of surgical intervention. We can consider these as actual and potential problems that patients may experience in the postoperative period. Obviously, for patients admitted for emergency surgery, some of these problems become more acute and require more urgent attention. Refer to Chapter 2 for additional material on the following topics, especially the problem-solving exercises.

Activity

Re-visit the CETL programme perioperative care resource at: http://www.cetl.org.uk/learning/perioperative-care/player.html (accessed December 2011).

This includes every stage of the perioperative period and postoperative observations.

Actual and potential problems postoperatively: principles of practice

Management of pain

Pain at some level is a consequence of surgery, the level of pain being dependent on the individual and their tolerance to pain and also to the type and extent of surgery experienced. The physical pain a nurse anticipates a patient will experience from surgery such as removal of the gall bladder via microscopic surgery may be different from the pain she will anticipate a patient may have following major thoracotomy and oesophagectomy. However, as we know, this is not how it may work out in the reality of practice. Consider this quote from McCaffrey (1979:3):

> ... *pain is a subjective experience – the person who helps the patient with pain cannot see or feel what is being treated. Further, psychosocial factors influence responses to pain and even the existence of pain to such an extent that two people exposed to the same potentially painful stimulus may react in opposite ways. Add to this the lack of knowledge about what causes the pain and what may relieve it. Unsurprisingly, the result often is one of disagreement among health professionals and between practitioner and the patient with pain.*

Management of fluid and electrolyte balance

If a patient has had major surgery, it is likely that he/she will have an intravenous infusion postoperatively in order to replace fluid loss and also prevent dehydration when fluid intake may be restricted and the patient may also not be eating immediately. This requires careful monitoring in terms of the prescribed regimen and for any signs of inflammation at the site of the cannula

(Scales 2008). Many patients will also be receiving medications via this infusion. See Box 9.5 for good practice to reduce infection in intravenous therapy. This guidance, however, is for qualified nurses, but if you are a member of the nursing team caring for a patient with an infusion postoperatively, you will undertake many observations related to this good practice alongside your mentor.

Management of postoperative nausea and vomiting

Postoperative nausea and vomiting (PONV) is also a problem for some patients and can cause stress, discomfort and additional pain (Gilmour 2010). Patients may be responding to the type of anaesthetic given during surgery, postoperative pain or the postoperative pain relief itself. Whatever the cause, it requires immediate response from nurses, something that Jolley (2000) found did not always happen. A more recent audit undertaken by DeLeskey (2009:141) examined whether or not 'best practice based on best available evidence for the management and treatment of PONV' was taking place. She found that change in practice was required in a number of areas, based on the six criteria she had selected for the audit (see Box 9.6).

Activity

Given that McCaffrey wrote this in 1979 (second edition of her classic work from 1972), does her observation still resonate with today's clinical practice? How often have you heard qualified nurses say to patients 'but you can't be in pain, you had pain relief 2 hours ago and are not due any more for another 2 hours at least' or the discussion between nurses on the dangers of patients becoming addicted to strong pain relief?

Discuss with your mentor their views on pain management. Consider the various ways in which patients cope with pain in your placement area and consider what the main differences involved in the surgery itself, the medication prescribed and the patient's concerns about pain relief were.

If you can obtain a copy of either McCaffrey's 1972 or 1979 book *Nursing Management of the Patient with Pain*, consider how her assertions on all aspects of pain management have changed over time. Obviously some of the medication has changed and there is additional research evidence available.

Assessing a patient's pain and managing the pain by various means is one of the main roles of the nurse postoperatively (see Ch. 2).

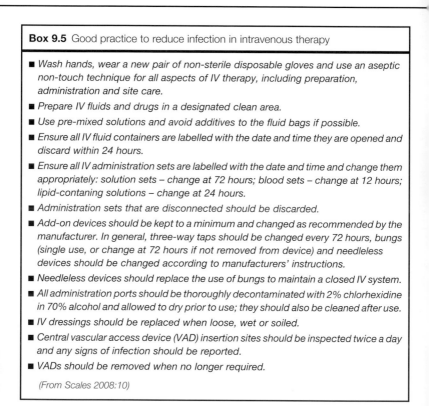

Box 9.5 Good practice to reduce infection in intravenous therapy

- *Wash hands, wear a new pair of non-sterile disposable gloves and use an aseptic non-touch technique for all aspects of IV therapy, including preparation, administration and site care.*
- *Prepare IV fluids and drugs in a designated clean area.*
- *Use pre-mixed solutions and avoid additives to the fluid bags if possible.*
- *Ensure all IV fluid containers are labelled with the date and time they are opened and discard within 24 hours.*
- *Ensure all IV administration sets are labelled with the date and time and change them appropriately: solution sets – change at 72 hours; blood sets – change at 12 hours; lipid-contaning solutions – change at 24 hours.*
- *Administration sets that are disconnected should be discarded.*
- *Add-on devices should be kept to a minimum and changed as recommended by the manufacturer. In general, three-way taps should be changed every 72 hours, bungs (single use, or change at 72 hours if not removed from device) and needleless devices should be changed according to manufacturers' instructions.*
- *Needleless devices should replace the use of bungs to maintain a closed IV system.*
- *All administration ports should be thoroughly decontaminated with 2% chlorhexidine in 70% alcohol and allowed to dry prior to use; they should also be cleaned after use.*
- *IV dressings should be replaced when loose, wet or soiled.*
- *Central vascular access device (VAD) insertion sites should be inspected twice a day and any signs of infection should be reported.*
- *VADs should be removed when no longer required.*

(From Scales 2008:10)

Activity

Discuss with your mentor what the current practice is for the management of patients who experience postoperative nausea and vomiting. Use the criteria in Box 9.6 as the basis for this discussion. Observe during your care of postoperative patients how many patients experience nausea and vomiting postoperatively and how it was managed by the surgical team.

Obtain a copy of Jolley (2001) (see References). Read it prior to starting your clinical placement. The article includes a number of 'Time Out' questions for the reader as part of continuing professional development. These include some questions related to risk factors and use of antiemetics. Try to answer the questions while reading the article. (If you subscribe to this journal, it also enables you to access a number of resources online which are related to surgical nursing in general).

Box 9.6 Six criteria to determine best practice in management and treatment of PONV

1. *PONV risk factors are identified and documented before surgery.*
2. *PONV risk factors are communicated to the anaesthetic/surgical team before surgery.*
3. *Appropriate PONV treatment is ordered to be given as needed postoperatively.*
4. *Appropriate PONV prophylaxis is administered as indicated by risk factors.*
5. *Routine assessment for PONV occurs postoperatively.*
6. *Appropriate PONV rescue treatment is initiated as needed.*

(From DeLeskey 2009:141)

The management of postoperative nausea and vomiting requires the involvement of the whole surgical team. Ensuring accurate recording of any vomiting together with observation of volume, colour, frequency and timing, however, is the responsibility of the nurse in the team, as is reassuring patients and relieving any distress they may experience. Ensuring you are aware of the evidence-based risk factors as well as the management of PONV enables you to enhance your nursing care of patients in the perioperative period. It is important to note that every patient and various surgical procedures will require a specific response and management, some of which are considered in the case studies in Section 3.

Management of nutrition

Depending on the type of surgery a patient undergoes, as well as their nutritional status when admitted to hospital, managing postoperative nutrition needs is an essential part of a nurse's role. It has been found that many elderly patients, for example, experience malnourishment during a stay in hospital, due in part to a lack of risk assessment or adequate monitoring of what they are eating (see RCN (2009) for an excellent guide to nutrition and older people).

Field and Bjarnason (2002:42) point out the importance of preoperative nutritional assessment and nurses' actions required for patients after abdominal surgery:

> *Nutritional assessment of ill patients anticipating major surgery is crucial, as deterioration of nutritional status is one of the key factors in surgical outcome. It is important, therefore, to obtain on admission weight, height and BMI [body mass index] score. This assessment can highlight those patients who are underweight and vulnerable on admission. This simple assessment can alert the surgeon to potential postoperative problems. The help and advice of the dietician or nutrition team can then be sought at an early stage.*

Activity

Obtain a copy of Field and Bjarnason (2002) and compare the practice on your placement with that in the article. Ensuring adequate nutritional intake is as important for day surgery or ambulatory care as it is for major surgery, either planned or emergency.

After major surgery, many patients return to the ward with an intravenous infusion in place in order to ensure adequate and appropriate fluid and electrolyte replacement as well as nutrients essential for postoperative healing and nutrition. The British Association of Parenteral and Enteral Nutrition has developed guidelines for intravenous fluid therapy for adult surgical patients, which includes some basic information regarding the links between physiology and management of patients perioperatively and evidence-based guidance on postoperative fluid and nutrition management (see http://www.bapen.org.uk/pdfs/bapen_pubs/giftasup.pdf (accessed December 2011)).

Management of infection control

Infection control issues have been discussed in Chapters 1–4 in relation to preparation prior to practice placement experience. It is recommended that you re-visit that section as well as the Nursing and Midwifery Council (NMC) essential skills cluster on infection prevention and control.

Postoperatively, the prevention of infection becomes a major nursing management task. It is directly linked to the management of wounds and wound care, but we also need to consider it in the broader context of hospital-acquired infections.

Depending on the type of surgery, you will see many different kinds of wounds, a variety of wound closure techniques, some with wound drains, and a variety of different wound dressings. These are known as surgical wounds, i.e. they are deliberate incisions in the skin which also impact on underlying structures and are usually performed in a clean environment where asepsis is maintained at all times (Pudner 2010). Wound care management postoperatively is aimed at promoting healing and

> **Box 9.7** Principles of surgical wound management
>
> ■ *To achieve healing of the wound.*
> ■ *To avoid complications, e.g. infection.*
> ■ *To achieve good pain control.*
> ■ *To ensure a cosmetically acceptable scar.*
> ■ *To allow the individual to return to a normal lifestyle as soon as possible.*
> *(From Pudner 2010:51)*

preventing infection (Gibson 2006), and Pudner (2010) identifies five principles of surgical wound management (see Box 9.7).

Examples of different kinds of suturing techniques and drains can be seen in Figures 9.1–9.6.

Activity

During your clinical placement, make a list of all the types of wound closure techniques you have seen and ask your mentor if you can first observe the removal of sutures/clips/drains, then gain experience in undertaking this yourself.

When to remove these is dependent on the surgeon's practice and/or the healing progress made by the patient.

Paper to read prior to placement:

Chapter 5 in Pudner (2010) (see References for further information. It includes an explanation of the knowledge of physiology and how the skin works, which is essential to an understanding of wound healing and infection prevention.

Subcuticular

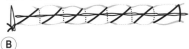

(A)

Continuous over-and-over

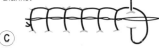

(B)

Blanket

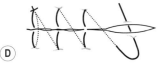

(C)

Continuous mattress

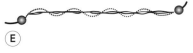

(D)

Subcuticular Prolene™ suture and

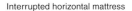

(E)

Fig 9.1 Types of continuous suturing techniques (reproduced from Pudner (2010) with permission)

Interrupted over-and-over

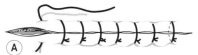

(A)

Interrupted vertical mattress

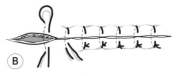

(B)

Interrupted horizontal mattress

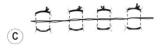

(C)

Fig 9.2 Types of interrupted suturing techniques (reproduced from Pudner (2010) with permission)

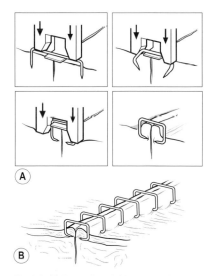

(A)

(B)

Fig 9.3 (A) Formation of skin staples. (B) Skin staples in situ (reproduced with permission of Ethicon Ltd)

A question often asked is: How do we know if a patient has a wound infection? Reilly (2002) offers the following definition, citing Emmerson et al (1993):

> *A wound infection should have either a purulent discharge in, or exuding from, the wound, or a painful erythema indicative of cellulitis. Infection should also be considered to be present when there is a fever (>38°C), tenderness, oedema and an extending margin of erythema, or the patient is still receiving active treatment for a wound which has discharged pus.*

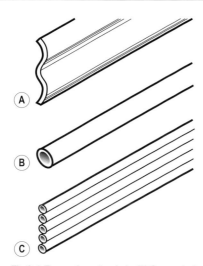

Fig 9.4 Types of passive drain: (A) Corrugated; (B) Penrose; (C) Yeats (reproduced from Pudner (2010) with permission)

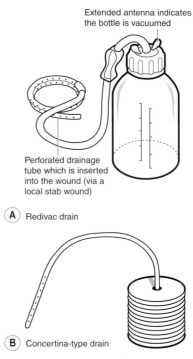

Extended antenna indicates the bottle is vacuumed

Perforated drainage tube which is inserted into the wound (via a local stab wound)

(A) Redivac drain

(B) Concertina-type drain

Fig 9.5 Types of active drain: (A) Redivac; (B) Concertina type (reproduced from Pudner (2010) with permission)

It is important that students can undertake aseptic technique, regardless of what type of clinical placement they are undertaking. Watch the video of this technique at the CETL website: http://www.cetl.org.uk/learning/aseptic-dressing-technique/player.html (accessed December 2011).

You may also have similar skills videos at your university – check out the information on your virtual learning environment (such as BlackBoard).

Of course, with many patients now being discharged home from hospital earlier than in the past and after any kind of surgery, the role of the hospital nurse in removal of sutures has altered because this role now belongs to the community health nurse. If you are following a patient pathway or placement learning experience where one of the perioperative areas is your main base or hub, it is a good idea to discuss with your mentor the possibility of visiting a patient

you have been caring for once they are discharged home (see Ch. 10).

Personal cleansing and dressing

Personal cleansing and dressing are very important for all patients, in particular the need for correct and appropriate skin care postoperatively. Many patients undergoing surgery are elderly and therefore have additional needs that younger patients don't have.

The symposium paper by Deshi (2010) offers an insight into some of the issues facing the care of elderly

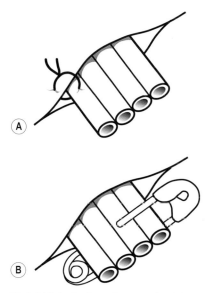

Fig 9.6 Methods of securing a passive drain in place: (A) Yeats drain secured in place with a suture; (B) Yeats drain secured in place by a safety pin (reproduced from Pudner (2010) with permission)

patients with co-morbidities (multiple diseases) and weak physiological strength. The paper also focuses on the value of a multidisciplinary approach to caring for an older person undergoing surgery.

 Activity

Obtain a copy of this paper online and consider its findings for patients in hospital and in the community:

http://www.rcpe.ac.uk/journal/issue/journal_40_4/dhesi.pdf (accessed December 2011).

Older patients, especially those who have multiple health problems, are at risk of developing pressure sores as well, especially if they do not mobilise quickly following surgery. Their skin may be less strong than when they were younger and they may also be on medication which may add to the problem. A preoperative assessment will identify those patients at risk.

Care of the mouth is also important, especially if patients are unable to eat or drink postoperatively, and there is a potential for mouth infections to occur. Some postoperative medications can also cause a dry mouth, especially steroids or oxygen therapy.

Other general personal cleansing and dressing issues involve different cultural and religious needs in relation to postoperative care, and maintaining the dignity of the patient.

A useful document has been published by the Association for Perioperative Practice (AfPP) on this very topic (AfPP 2007). This includes guidance on skin assessment in the perioperative environment, including assessing for cyanosis in darker skin.

Mobilising

Movement is encouraged postoperatively according to the nature of the surgery and the patient pathways for certain health problems (conditions). Apart from the potential to develop pressure ulcers and chest infections, there is the added potential problem of the development of deep vein thrombosis and/or a pulmonary embolism (see the National Institute for Health and Clinical Excellence (NICE 2010) guidelines at: http://www.nice.org.uk/CG92). Patients are mobilised according to the nature of their surgery: an elderly patient, for example, with a fractured femur who has been to theatre for a 'pin and plate' will be mobilised very differently to someone who has had an above-the-knee amputation or a total hip replacement.

Activity

Consider the practice in your clinical placement with regards to mobilisation of patients postoperatively. If it is an orthopaedic ward, for example, make a list of all the various types of surgery or care given to patients and discuss with your mentor how each patient is normally mobilised after surgery.

Elimination needs

There is a change in patterns of elimination postoperatively, and even patients who have been admitted for ambulatory or day care surgery may stay in hospital because they are unable to pass urine postoperatively and may need catheterisation.

Most patients returning from the operating theatre do not have a catheter in place, but for some types of surgery this is an automatic practice. Examples are major gynaecology surgery, major abdominal surgery or genitourinary surgery.

It is important for patients to pass urine postoperatively to avoid being catheterised and to prevent risk of urinary tract infection.

Urinary retention can be caused by opioids given for postoperative pain, as they act on the bladder's voiding reflex (Kitcatt 2010). They can also cause constipation because they 'delay gastric emptying and reduce the propulsive contractions in the gut' (Kitcatt 2010:115).

Paralytic ileus is also a potential problem for patients, especially after major abdominal surgery or surgery to the gastrointestinal tract. It is a term used to describe stasis within the bowel. When the bowel is operated on, the nerve pathways are interrupted, which can result in the temporary loss of peristalsis (Felstead 2007). This means that patients are unable to eat or drink postoperatively as planned due to their bowel not working properly. In cases where

there is a paralytic ileus diagnosed, 'the surgical team will listen for bowel sounds on a daily basis and usually commence the patient on small amounts of water gradually building up to free fluids and full diet over a number of days' (Felstead 2007:155).

 Activity

Holland et al (2008) cite Brown's (2002) criteria for determining successful outcomes of postoperative care, which are given in Box 9.8.

Depending on your placement, consider the variance from this standardised list of criteria and what care took place to achieve these outcomes. Discuss as a learning goal with your mentor.

Box 9.8 Determining successful outcomes of care postoperatively

1. The patient is free from pain and discomfort, as shown by verbal expression and participation in physical activities and ability to rest and sleep.
2. The fluid intake and electrolyte concentrations are normal for the patient.
3. The patient is taking a nutritionally balanced diet.
4. Urinary and bowel elimination are re-established and normal for the patient.
5. The patient is ambulatory, active and participating in care.
6. The incision is clean, dry and intact.
7. Vital signs are normal for the patient.
8. No manifestations of complications are present.

> **Box 9.8** Determining successful outcomes of care postoperatively— cont'd
>
> 9. The patient and family demonstrate an understanding of the required care during convalescence and the resources available.
>
> *(From Holland et al 2008, citing Brown 2002:190)*

For the majority of patients, this is a normal pattern in terms of measuring a successful postoperative period. Those who develop some of the complications mentioned in this section recover from them, but obviously there are occasions when patients die postoperatively. This may be due to some postoperative complications or to a previously undiagnosed problem which may have led to a cardiac arrest, for example, either in the operating theatre or when returned to the ward.

All surgery carries risk, but if the preoperative assessment has been effective in identifying potential problems and the postoperative care has been managed well and underpinned by an evidence base, then these risks are minimised. The majority of patients are then discharged home from hospital.

Discharge home from hospital

In brief, as this is discussed fully in Chapter 10, planned discharge begins prior to or on admission of the patient for either minor or major surgery. Other agencies may well have to be contacted and follow-up appointments organised. Patients are now discharged home into the care of their GP and the district nursing team. The reduction in hospital stays postoperatively has meant a shift in what happens to patients and their care, with community nurses taking over many postoperative care procedures and continuing to observe for postoperative complications which can still occur and may result in the patient being re-admitted to hospital.

Summary

This chapter has given you a brief insight into the postoperative care of the patient. Given the number and variety of surgical interventions, the presentation has been mainly generic. More explicit examples are explored in Section 3.

Many of the issues discussed here will support your development and achievement of the NMC Essential Skills and Standards for becoming 'fit for practice' as a nurse. We return to these in Section 4 when we look at future learning needs, testing what you have learnt through this book and also looking forward to other placements and what you can continue in your ongoing record of achievement (NMC 2010).

References

Allen, D., 2005. Sensory receptors and sense organs. In: Montague, S., Watson, R., Herbert, R.A. (Eds.), Physiology for nursing practice, 3rd ed. Elsevier, Edinburgh: 133–148.

Allvin, R., Berg, K., Idvall, E., Nilsson, U., 2006. Postoperative recovery: a concept analysis. Journal of Advanced Nursing 57 (5), 552–558.

Amos, A., Waugh, A., 2007. Caring for the person having surgery. In: Brooker, C., Waugh, A. (Eds.), Foundations of nursing practice. Mosby, Edinburgh: 681–702.

Association for Perioperative Practice, 2007. Respecting cultural diversity in the perioperative setting. AfPP, Harrogate.

Bell, L., Duffy, A., 2009. Pain assessment and management in surgical nursing: a literature review. British Journal of Nursing 18 (3), 153–156.

Bennallick, M., King, D., 2009. Infection prevention and control, essential skills 4.1. In: Endacott, R., Jevon, P., Cooper, S. (Eds.), Clinical nursing skills – core and advanced. Oxford University Press, Oxford.

Brown, A., 2002. The patient undergoing surgery. In: Walsh, M. (Ed.), Watson's clinical nursing and related sciences, sixth ed. Baillière Tindall/Royal College of Nursing, London: 65–192.

DeLeskey, K., 2009. The implementation of evidence-based practice for the prevention/management of post-operative nausea and vomiting. International Journal of Evidence-Based Healthcare 7, 140–144.

Department of Health, 2010. The Health and Social Care Act 2008: code of practice on the prevention and control of infections and related guidance. DH, London.

Deshi, J., 2010. Improving outcomes in older people undergoing elective surgery (symposium review). Journal of the Royal College of Physicians 40, 348–353.

Emmerson, A.M., Ayliffe, G.A.J., Casewell, M.W., et al., 1993. National prevalence survey of hospital acquired infections. Journal of Hospital Infection 24, 69–76.

Endacott, R., Jevon, P., Cooper, S., 2009. Clinical Nursing skills – Core and Advanced. Oxford University Press, Oxford.

Felstead, I., 2007. Surgery of the lower gastrointestinal tract. In: McArthur-Rouse, F., Prosser, S. (Eds.), Assessing and managing the acutely ill adult surgical patient. Blackwell, Oxford: 145–157.

Field, J., Bjarnason, K., 2002. Feeding patients after abdominal surgery. Nursing Standard 16 (48), 41–44.

Gibson, C., 2006. The patient facing surgery. In: Alexander, M., Fawcett, J.N., Runciman, P.J. (Eds.), Nursing practice hospital and home: the adult, 3rd ed. Churchill Livingstone, Edinburgh.

Gibson, C., Magowan, R., 2011. The patient undergoing surgery. In: Brooker, C., Nicol, M. (Eds.), Alexander's nursing practice, 4th ed. Churchill Livingstone, Edinburgh.

Gilmour, D., 2010. Perioperative care. In: Pudner, R. (Ed.), Nursing the surgical patient, 3rd ed. Baillière Tindall, Edinburgh: 17–34.

Gray, A., Hart, M., Dalrymple, K., Davies, T., 2008. Promoting safe transfusion practice: right blood, right patient, right time. British Journal of Nursing 17 (13), 812–817.

Heikkinen, K., Salantera, S., Kettu, M., Taittonen, M., 2005. Prostatectomy patients' postoperative pain assessment in the recovery room. Journal of Advanced Nursing 52 (6), 592–600.

Holland, K., Jenkins, J., Solomon, J., Whittam, S., 2008. Applying the Roper, Logan and Tierney model in practice. Churchill Livingstone, Edinburgh.

Hughes, S., 2004. Principles of post-operative patient care. Nursing Standard 19 (5), 43–51.

Huskinson, W., Lloyd, H., 2009. Oral health in hospitalised patients: assessment and hygiene. Nursing Standard 23 (36), 43–47.

Johnstone, C.C., Rattray, J., Myers, L., 2007. Physiological risk factors, early warning scoring systems and organizational changes. British Association of Critical

Care Nurses, Nursing in Critical Care 12 (5), 219–224.

Jolley, S., 2000. Post-operative nausea and vomiting: a survey of nurses' knowledge. Nursing Standard 14 (23), 32–34.

Jolley, S., 2001. Managing postoperative nausea and vomiting. Nursing Standard 15 (40), 47–52.

Kitcatt, S., 2010. Concepts of pain and the surgical patient. In: Pudner, R. (Ed.), Nursing the surgical patient, 3rd ed. Baillière Tindall, Edinburgh.

McCaffrey, M., 1979. Nursing management of the patient with pain, 2nd ed. J B Lippincott, Philadelphia.

NHS Forth Valley, 2009. Management of adult patients with diabetes undergoing elective surgery. NHS Forth Valley, Falkirk.

NHS Quality Improvement Scotland, 2004. Postoperative pain management. NHS Scotland, Edinburgh.

Nursing and Midwifery Council, 2010. Standards for pre-registration nursing education. NMC, London.

Oldham, J., Sinclair, L., Hendry, C., 2009. Right blood, right patient, right care: safe transfusion practice. British Journal of Nursing 18 (5), 312–320.

Preston, R., Flynn, D., 2010. Key points from a review of the evidence: observations in acute care: evidence-based approach to patient safety. British Journal of Nursing 19 (7), 442–447.

Pudner, R. (Ed.), 2010. Nursing the surgical patient, 3rd ed. Baillière Tindall, Edinburgh.

Reilly, J., 2002. Evidence-based surgical wound care on a surgical wound infection. British Journal of Nursing 11 (16), S4–S12.

Royal College of Nursing, 2009. Nutrition and older people: essential guide. RCN, London.Online. Available at: http://rcn-library.rcn.org.uk/uhtbin/cgisirsi/0/0/0/

5?searchdata1=a318466{001}/ (accessed December 2011).

Royal College of Nursing, 2011. Promoting older people's oral health: essential guide. RCN, London. Online. Available at: http://nursingstandard.rcnpublishing.co.uk/shared/media/pdfs/OralHealth2011.pdf (accessed December 2011).

Scales, K., 2008. Intravenous therapy: a guide to good practice. British Journal of Nursing 17 (19), S4–S12.

Scottish Intercollegiate Guidelines Network, 2002. Postoperative management in adults. SIGN, Edinburgh. Online. Available at: http://www.sign.ac.uk/pdf/sign77.pdf (accessed December 2011).

Smith, B., Hardy, D., 2007. Discharge criteria: 'just in case'. Journal of Perioperative Practice 17 (3), 102 104–107.

Torrance, C., Serginson, E., 1999. Surgical nursing, twelfth ed. Baillière Tindall/Royal College of Nursing, London.

Wicker, P., Cox, F., 2010. Patient during recovery. In: Wicker, P., O'Neil, J. (Eds.), Caring for the perioperative patient, 2nd ed. Wiley-Blackwell, Oxford.

Further reading

European Society of Regional Anaesthesia, Postoperative pain management – good clinical practice. General recommendations and principles for successful pain management. (undated) Online. Available at: http://www.esraeurope.org/PostoperativePainManagement.pdf (accessed May 2011).

Hindle, A., Coates, A., 2011. Nursing care of older people. Oxford University Press, Oxford.

Holland, K., Hogg, C., 2010. Cultural awareness in nursing and healthcare. Arnold, London.

Hughes, A., 2009. Pre- and post-operative assessment and care: essential skills. In: Endacott, R., Jevon, P., Cooper, S. (Eds.), Clinical nursing skills – core and advanced. Oxford University Press, Oxford.

National Clinical Guideline Centre, 2010. Venous thromboembolism: reducing the risk of venous thromboembolism (deep vein thrombosis and pulmonary embolism) in patients admitted to hospital. NCGC, The Royal College of Physicians, London. Online. Available at: http://www.nice.org.uk/nicemedia/live/12695/47920/47920.pdf (accessed December 2011).

Razouk, K., Harrison, L., Taljard, F., 2010. Perioperative management of diabetic patients undergoing surgery. NHS Lanarkshire. Online. Available at: http://www.pdc.nhsscotland.com/PracticeandLearning/PoliciesGuidelines/Policies%20and%20Guidelines/Periop%20Mgmt%20Diabetic%20Patients%20Undergoing%20Surgery.pdf (accessed June 2011).

Websites

RCN guidance for improving transfusion practice: http://www.rcn.org.uk/__data/assets/pdf_file/0009/78615/002306.pdf (accessed December 2011).

Insulin pump therapy (registered users only – RCN membership or a journal subscription): http://nursingstandard.rcnpublishing.co.uk/guides/booklets-and-guides/insulin-pump-therapy (accessed December 2011).

NHS Forth Valley publications: http://www.nhsforthvalley.com/publications/ (accessed December 2011).

NICE guidance on perioperative nutritional support in adults – oral nutrition, enteral tube feeding and parenteral nutrition: http://www.nice.org.uk/nicemedia/live/10978/29981/29981.pdf (accessed December 2011).

Healthcare-associated infections (CETL online site). This session offers explanations by patients and carers of what having a healthcare-associated infection meant to them and how they managed: http://www.cetl.org.uk/learning/healthcare_associated_infections/player.html (accessed December 2011).

NHS Local: Better Health Together information website. This site offers a range of resources for people and their carers (lay and professional) and includes video material of patients talking about some of the issues affecting them. There are also explanations about a wide range of conditions in the section on My Health: http://nhslocal.nhs.uk/my-health/conditions/b/pressure-ulcers/all (accessed December 2011).

10   Going home from hospital

CHAPTER AIMS

- To enable the student to gain an understanding of patients' discharge home from hospital following surgery
- To gain an overview of the integration of care delivery and continuity of care experience
- To gain an overview of key health and social care professionals responsible for care of the patient following discharge home after surgery

Introduction

Going home from hospital is a welcome event for the majority of patients, where they can be assured of support from their families and a range of services. For others, it is a more worrying event, especially if they live alone and may have less access to services they might require. For the majority of patients, regardless of their level of support, there will be concerns about how they are going to manage after surgery. This concern will, of course, be dependent on the kind of surgery and, most importantly, what kind of diagnosis may have been the outcome (e.g. if a patient has undergone surgery for removal of a cancerous tumour, worry over whether it has all been removed or not). Psychological care and effective communication are two very important areas where the nurse has to develop skills, and as a student nurse you will be assessed in these areas as part of your 'fitness for practice' Nursing and Midwifery Council (NMC) (2010) standards (see Box 10.1 for examples of relevant competencies to be achieved).

Preparation for discharge from hospital

Preparation for a patient's discharge from hospital is a multidisciplinary team effort which is coordinated in most situations by the nurse. This person is referred to as the ward-based care coordinator in the Department of Health (DH) (2003) guidance. As can be seen in the DH (2003) principles, it is implicit in any policy to ensure that discharge planning should be co-ordinated by one person.

The DH (2003:46) sees this as part of 'co-ordinating the patient journey' and identifies the following key principles

---

Box 10.1 NMC (2010) Standards

Domain 2 – Communication and Interpersonal Skills

2.2. All nurses must use a range of communication skills and technologies to support person-centred care and enhance quality and safety. They must ensure people receive all the information they need in a language and manner that allows them to make informed choices and share decision making. They must recognise when language interpretation or other communication support is needed and know how to obtain it.

Domain 3 – Nursing Practice and Decision Making

3.3. All nurses must ascertain and respond to the physical, social and psychological needs of people, groups and communities. They must then plan, deliver and evaluate safe, competent, person-centred care in partnership with them, paying special attention to changing health needs during different life stages, including progressive illness and death, loss and bereavement.

For students who have to achieve competencies according to the NMC 2004 standards, there are similar experiences to be achieved (please refer to your practice assessment documents for comparative competencies).

---

underpinning this aspect of effective discharge and transfer of care policy:

- *Discharge is a process and not an isolated event. It has to be planned for at the earliest opportunity between the primary, hospital and social care organisations, ensuring that patients and their carer(s) understand and are able to contribute to care planning decisions as appropriate.*
- *The process of discharge planning should be co-ordinated by a named person who has responsibility for coordinating all stages of the patient's progress. This involves liaison with the pre-admission case coordinator in the community at the earliest opportunity and the transfer of those responsibilities on discharge.*
- *Staff should work within a framework of integrated multidisciplinary and multiagency team working to manage all aspects of the discharge process.*

Activity

Consider these three principles and ask your mentor if you can be involved in the discharge experience of a patient's journey from hospital to home. Set out what your main learning objectives are in relation to the experience and use this as a goal for your expected learning outcomes in the placement. This could involve the discharge of a patient from a day care unit or a ward.

To help with this, obtain a copy of the article by Goodman (2010) (see References), which considers the importance of planning for discharge from hospital.

The nurse's role in discharging patients home from hospital

If we use the idea of the nurse as the ward-based care coordinator, the DH (2003) document states that 'this is an important, highly skilled role and requires an experienced practitioner who has a good understanding of discharge planning'. Key tasks considered to be important to this role are given in Box 10.2. The report suggested that this role could be enhanced to include nurse-led discharge.

You may come across patients who decide that they no longer want to stay in hospital and choose this against medical advice. It is important to consider whether the patient 'understands the risks they are taking in discharging themselves' or whether in fact they are 'not competent to understand the risks associated with discharge due to his or her medical condition' or the same but 'due to mental health problems' DH (2003).

The DH (2010) has published a good practice toolkit for organisations to ensure best practice in discharge planning. You can access this for general information at: http://www.dh.gov.uk/en/Publicationsandstatistics/Publications/PublicationsPolicyAnd Guidance/DH_113950 (accessed July 2011).

Oakley (2010) also sets out the criteria for discharge of a patient following day surgery which can be used as an aide-memoire for checking what needs to happen prior to the patient going home. These criteria are given in Box 10.3.

Box 10.2 Care coordinator key tasks

- *Coordinate patient assessment, care planning and daily review of the care pathway.*
- *Discuss with the patient a potential transfer/discharge date usually within 24 hours of admission and recorded in the patient's notes.*
- *Ensure that timely referrals are made, results are received and any delays are followed up.*
- *Identify, involve and inform the patient about all aspects of care planning, ensuring that the special needs of young carers are identified.*
- *Engage the carer and make arrangements for carer assessment.*
- *If appropriate, make arrangements to see the carer separately regarding their own needs.*
- *Keep the patient's documentation up to date.*
- *Liaise with and work as an integral member of the interdisciplinary team and care management services.*
- *Liaise with specialist nursing services and other specialist services as appropriate.*
- *Finalise the transfer/discharge arrangements 48 hours before discharge and confirm with the patient and carer/family.*
- *On day of transfer/discharge, ensue the patient's condition remains as expected and confirm follow-up arrangements.*

  (From DH 2003:55)

Box 10.3 Criteria for discharge after day surgery

- *The patient should be alert and orientated.*
- *The patient should tolerate diet and fluids, i.e. not vomiting.*
- *The patient should have voided urine.*
- *The patient should be comfortable and mobile, i.e. should be pain free.*
- *Baseline observations must be satisfactory.*
- *Wound checks must be satisfactory, i.e. the dressing is dry, there is no fresh bleeding.*
- *Any follow-up appointments (if required) should be arranged.*
- *Any mobility aids such as crutches (if required) should be supplied.*
- *The patient must have a discharge letter for their GP.*
- *Verbal and written discharge information should be given.*
- *Any medication to take home (if required) must be given.*

(From Oakley 2010:41)

Practice placement learning pathways (hub and spoke placements) and discharge planning and implementation

As a student, it is important to be able to gain experience in this process in any context. As discussed in earlier chapters, given the importance also of understanding the patient's journey during admission for surgery and ongoing care during the perioperative period, it is an excellent opportunity to gain experience with members of the multidisciplinary health and social care services and learn about their part in the discharge of patients from hospital. Examples of members of the multidisciplinary team who may be involved in discharge planning and implementation are:

- social services: social worker
- occupational therapist
- district nurses
- dietician
- pharmacist
- specialist nurses, e.g. pain management, breast cancer, diabetic, cardiac rehabilitation nurses
- GP.

Activity

Discuss with your mentor which members of the team you would like to talk with to find out their role in the discharge of patients from hospital after surgery. Obtain support to contact those who are involved with patients in your placement.

The type of surgery a patient has undergone as well as their general health state will determine who is involved in their discharge home from hospital. Liaison at all times with family members or carers is essential. One of the key criteria is ensuring that there is someone to collect the patient, or there is transport organised, and that there will be someone to look after the patient when they arrive at their destination. For those patients in care homes, it is essential that the transfer from hospital is completed with essential notes/information about the surgery and the postoperative care given.

The nurse's role in the aftercare of the patient following discharge home from hospital (the first 2 weeks)

Once patients hasve been discharged following surgery, they are in the care of the health centre and their GP, together with the community nursing team. A written discharge summary will have been sent to the GP together with some kind of care transfer plan which will enable the essential continuity of care to be carried out. A follow-up appointment to check on the patient's progress will have been made with the patient's consultant surgeon and his/her team. If there is a discharge co-ordinator in charge of the patient's discharge, they will act as the main liaison with the relevant agencies involved in the community. Social services may be involved if the patient requires additional support: for example, if they live alone, a 'meals at home' service may have to be organised.

Given that patients' stay in hospital, even for major surgery, is now much shorter than in the past, patients can still require care that they would normally have had in hospital. In addition, some postoperative complications may still occur, and the community team will be vigilant in their observations with regards to these, working together with either the family or carer and, in some situations, care home staff.

Potential complications or problems could be:

- wound infection
- secondary haemorrhage (up to 10 days postoperatively)
- fistula formation (an abnormal track connecting two viscera, e.g. rectum and vagina (Pudner 2010:69))
- wound dehiscence (partial or complete separation of a surgically closed wound (Pudner 2010:69),

mainly abdominal wounds, and known as a 'burst abdomen')
- continuing postoperative pain.

Activity

As part of your placement experience, discuss with your mentor the possibility of talking to district nurses in the community about the way in which they manage these kinds of complications which may require re-admission of the patient to hospital. Make notes on each of them as part of your ongoing learning plans and also as revision notes should you have an examination or case study question as a summative assignment at university (see Section 4 for examples).

One of the tasks that nurses in the community now undertake is removal of sutures at the agreed postoperative period, and for many of you, developing skills in removing a variety of wound closure materials such as clips and sutures will be gained in your community placements rather than in a surgical one. It is imperative, however, that you become familiar with all kinds of techniques in this area in order to be able to answer patients' questions with regards to wound care following their discharge from hospital. This applies to both day care patients and those who have had major surgery.

Supporting the patient and their family following discharge home

If a patient has had major surgery, they will require emotional support as well as practical, especially if the diagnosis linked to the surgery was not favourable (e.g. cancer diagnosis). Often surgery may be a palliative short-term outcome to ensure an enhanced quality of life for the patient. This would have been discussed with them following surgery. They may need further surgery and/or chemotherapy and radiotherapy. Again, it is essential that you are aware of the possible outcomes of surgery, and your mentor can support your learning by enabling you to observe him/her discussing with patients some of the questions they may have in relation to such outcomes. Gaining permission of the patient is important in situations where confidentiality or sensitive issues are going to be discussed.

Patients discharged from hospital have access to the whole community multidisciplinary team. If you are undertaking a community placement, one of your opportunities for learning about caring for a patient undergoing surgery will be the reverse of someone on a surgical ward placement. Your mentors may already have a system in place where there is a 'swapping over' of students in order to ensure that you gain an overall experience of the patient journey.

Summary

Management of a patient's discharge home from hospital begins on their admission to hospital. NHS trusts and surgical wards have policies and procedures in place to ensure effective and continuous care of the patient, which includes liaising with family and carers who will be the main support for the patient when they arrive home.

Understanding the evidence base for effective discharge planning and management of the postoperative period following discharge is key to your successful learning of total patient care.

References

Department of Health, 2003. Discharge from hospital: pathway, process and practice. DH, London. Online. Available at: http://www.dh.gov.uk/en/Publicationsandstatistics/Publications/PublicationsPolicyAndGuidance/DH_4003252 (accessed July 2011).

Department of Health, 2010. Ready to go? Planning the discharge and the transfer of patients from hospital and intermediate care. DH, London.

Goodman, H., 2010. Discharge from hospital: the importance of planning. British Journal of Cardiac Nursing 5 (6), 274–279.

Nursing and Midwifery Council, 2010. Standards for pre-registration nursing education. NMC, London.

Oakley, M., 2010. Day surgery. In: Pudner, R. (Ed.), Nursing the surgical patient, 3rd ed. Baillière Tindall, Edinburgh: 35–44.

Pudner, R. (Ed.), 2010. Nursing the surgical patient, 3rd ed. Baillière Tindall, Edinburgh.

Further reading

European Society of Regional Anaesthesia and Pain Therapy (undated). Postoperative pain management. Online. Available at: http://www.esraeurope.org/PostoperativePainManagement.pdf.

Royal College of Nursing, 2010. Discharge planning; a summary of the Department of Health's guidance. Ready to go? Planning the discharge and the transfer of patients from hospital and intermediate care. RCN, London. Online. Available at: http://emergencynurse.rcnpublishing.co.uk/shared/media/pdfs/discharge.pdf (accessed July 2011).

Website

NHS Institute for Innovation and Improvement. This site offers a range of guidance documents related to discharge planning, including preoperative assessment, discharge planning following day surgery and discharge planning for people with complex needs: http://www.institute.nhs.uk/quality_and_service_improvement_tools/quality_and_service_improvement_tools/discharge_planning.html (accessed July 2011).

Section 3. The patient experience of undergoing surgery

In this section, we help you to integrate what is discussed in earlier chapters through a series of case studies, focusing on three different kinds of patient care experiences and underpinned by a research evidence base.

The case studies focus on the surgical journey and link to previous chapters through specific learning exercises during clinical placements. They also help you to understand the importance of a holistic approach to the patient journey. This includes the importance of your developing a knowledge base of both normal physiology and abnormal physiology as a result of surgery and postoperatively. The case studies also introduce you to ways in which you can meet your practice outcomes in the variety of clinical placements identified as 'surgical'.

11 Case study 1: caring for a patient in a day care unit

CHAPTER AIMS

- To enable you to reflect on prior learning from other chapters
- To explore in more detail, through a specific case study, the kind of surgical interventions you may come across in a day care unit
- To focus on the total patient care of a patient who may be admitted into a day care unit for surgery, from pre-admission to discharge home and care in the community
- To enable you to identify learning opportunities as well as meet your practice learning outcomes

Introduction

This chapter introduces you to a focused approach to the care of a patient in a day care unit. As this is a book about actual clinical placements, the focus is on what you can learn about specific patient care, and it brings together all the knowledge and skills you have learned in other sections of the book in order to make maximum use of learning in a day care unit placement.

Introduction to patient and clinical problem

Mr John Roberts, age 48, has been given an initial diagnosis by his GP as having an inguinal hernia. His medical history notes that he had been building an extension to his house which has required lifting heavy building materials. He has a visible swelling in his groin area.

Following a referral to a consultant surgeon at his local district general hospital, it has been decided that this problem needs to be addressed soon and that repair of this hernia can be undertaken as a day care patient.

Before we consider his perioperative care, it is important that you consider the diagnosis and the possible signs and symptoms Mr Roberts may be experiencing.

What is a hernia?

In broad terms, a hernia is a *'protrusion of an organ or part of an organ through a weak point or aperture in the surrounding structures'* (Waugh & Grant 2010:321). According to Waugh & Grant (2010), there are seven different types of hernia affecting different parts of the body and with different causes. These are:

- *inguinal hernia*
- *femoral hernia*
- *umbilical hernia*
- *incisional hernia*
- *hiatus hernia*
- *peritoneal hernia*
- *congenital diaphragmatic hernia.*

Activity

Find out where in the body each of these hernias occur and make notes of the specific definition of each.

You will likely find a definition for an inguinal hernia similar to that from Waugh and Grant (2010:321): *'The weak point is the inguinal canal, which contains the spermatic cord in the male and the round ligament in the female. It occurs more commonly in males than females'.*

A similar definition from Kurzer et al (2007:318) states that an inguinal hernia is where part of the small bowel has protruded through the abdominal wall and causes *'a swelling in the groin which appears on straining, lifting or standing'* and there may be *'pain or discomfort in association with the swelling'.*

In addition, access the NHS Choices website where you can see a video plus other information about the causes of hernia, possible outcomes and the procedures used to correct the problem:

http://www.nhs.uk/conditions/hernia/Pages/Introduction.aspx (accessed December 2011).

An excellent tool for decision making on appropriate treatment for a hernia is the NHS Choices Map of Medicine: http://www.nhs.uk/Conditions/Hernia/Pages/MapofMedicinepage.aspx (accessed July 2011).

Kurzer et al (2007) state that whereas in the past, many hernias were treated with a 'truss' (a device that held a pad firmly against the deep inguinal canal and prevented the hernia coming out), it is normal today to undertake a surgical repair which aims to *'eliminate the swelling, relieve discomfort and remove the risk of strangulation'* (2007:319).

One of the major complications of an untreated hernia is that known as a strangulated hernia, which is a surgical emergency due to the possible outcomes if left untreated. See Box 11.1 for an explanation and how it is treated.

Care and management of the patient in the perioperative period

Your surgical placement may well be in a day care unit. You will have prepared yourself for this experience (see Chs 1–4) and made contact with the ward/unit and your mentor. On arrival at the unit and on meeting your mentor, you will discuss what the expectations are with regards to your practice assessment documents, as well as defining your placement learning pathway or 'hub and spoke' experiences (see Ch. 3).

Remember, you can learn and undertake a wide range of skills if your main placement is in a day care unit and, in particular, you will achieve competencies in all four

---

Box 11.1 Strangulation of a hernia

This life-threatening complication presents with all the symptoms of intestinal obstruction, e.g. vomiting, severe abdominal pain, distension and absolute constipation. The patient rapidly becomes shocked, dehydrated and pyrexial. Diagnosis is made by history and clinical examination. A plain X-ray may identify the location and the associated distended loops of bowel. Rapid preparation for surgery is necessary and definitive therapy includes oxygen, opiate analgesics, IV correction of fluid and electrolyte balance, nasogastric aspiration and antibiotic administration. Surgery may well necessitate resection of the affected bowel and intensive nursing care will probably be required in the early postoperative period.

Activity

Read a physiology textbook and consider the anatomical structures involved in an inguinal hernia as well as the digestive system in general (e.g. see Kurzer et al 2007). Review your understanding of a strangulated hernia and emergency admission procedures.

Mr Roberts does not have a strangulated hernia and has been admitted for repair of his inguinal hernia via laparoscopic surgery (see Kurzer et al (2007) for an excellent description of the repair procedure and choices).

---

of the Nursing and Midwifery Council (NMC) domains (NMC 2010). Prior experience and what you have to achieve at this specific point in your programme will determine which skills you will need to practice as well as what knowledge you need to acquire to care for a wide ranging group of patients admitted for day care surgery.

Day care surgery has increased over the past decade (Oakley 2010) and there are many advantages to it, in particular *'avoiding unnecessary hospital stay … preference to have their aftercare at home rather than hospital, and minimal disruption of daily routine'* (2010:36).

Paper to read prior to placement:

Oakley M., (2010) Day Surgery. In: Pudner, R. (Ed.), Nursing the surgical patient, 3rd ed. Baillière Tindall, Edinburgh.

If you are in your final year of study and have to achieve evidence of leadership, management and team working, a day care unit is an ideal environment in which to gain experience in all three areas. Because of the variety of health problems that patients present with, it is an opportunity for you learn all about a wide range of conditions.

Pre-admission clinic

Mr Roberts will have been sent an appointment to attend the pre-admission clinic where a preoperative assessment will be carried out by members of the surgical team (which are becoming increasingly nurse led) (Oakley & Bratchell 2010). Re-visit Chapter 5 to identify the principles of preoperative assessment, the aim of which, according to Oakley and Bratchell (2010:4), is this:

Preoperative assessment aims to minimise patient risk by assessing fitness for surgery, provide information to facilitate informed choice, reduce anxiety about hospital admission and to improve the patient experience. It should take into account the physiological, psychological and social needs of the patient undergoing surgery.

Activity

Consider how a nursing model such as the Roper, Logan and Tierney model (Holland et al 2008) can be applied within a day care environment, especially in helping nurses to focus on the above definition of the aim of preoperative assessment. Use the patient assessment sheet found in Appendix 3 of Holland et al's (2008) book, which also includes a discharge summary assessment sheet. Compare this with any documentation used in your placement. The assessment schedule questions found in Appendix 4 of Holland et al (2008) is also helpful in the preoperative assessment process as it takes into account questions related to activities of living as well as the physical, psychological, sociocultural, environmental and politicoeconomic aspects of a person's needs.

See Box 5.1 in Chapter 5 for the objectives of a preoperative assessment.

During Mr Roberts 's assessment it was clear that he was fit for surgery and the anaesthetic, his wife who accompanied him would be his main contact point and would be collecting him after his surgery. Pre-operative instructions were also given to him and information about when to call the Unit to check any concerns prior to his given date of admission as well as pre-operative preparation information such as not having anything to eat from midnight the night before, can still drink water/tea or coffee (minimal mil) up to 6.30 am if going to theatre in the morning. If an afternoon admission he can have a very light breakfast (tea and toast) before 7.30 am and only drink water/tea/coffee as before until 10 am. This kind of instruction is common throughout NHS instructions to patients. e.g. http://www.thh.nhs.uk/Patients/Daycase/daycase.htm (accessed July 2nd 2011).

Informed consent was also obtained and information sheets related to his inguinal hernia repair should also be available for him to take home. He may also have been asked to complete a preoperative assessment questionnaire which would be part of the preoperative assessment to identify health needs, allergies, physical problems and any post-discharge needs (see Chapter 1 - Appendix in Pudner R 2010) Mr Roberts is not a smoke so did not require instructions regarding not smoking 24 hours prior to surgery.

On the ward

Mr Roberts was asked to attend the day care unit 4 weeks after his pre-admission assessment. On arrival, he was greeted by the day care unit receptionist who checked his name on the surgical list for the day and his appointment letter. His admission was at 8 am.

As Mr Roberts is being admitted for his surgery as a day care patient, refer to Chapter 6 to help you write a plan of care from his arrival on

Activity

Imagine that, under supervision of your mentor, you are to admit Mr Roberts, stay with him during his surgery and look after him when he returns to the unit until he goes home. As well as assessing any needs and checking he understands what is going to happen (so that his consent is informed), you need to check if he has brought any medications, his pyjamas, dressing gown/slippers (if needed) and, most importantly, you must check his contact details and who is picking him up later in the day.

Have another look at the Hillingdon Hospitals website for examples of hospital information for day care patients:

http://www.thh.nhs.uk/Patients/ Daycase/daycase.htm (accessed July 2011).

the ward until he goes to the operating theatre.

It is important to keep reassuring Mr Roberts and encourage him to ask questions if he is at all worried or stressed about going to theatre and having an anaesthetic. An NMC domain competence that you can achieve in such a situation (among many) is that of communication and interpersonal skills (NMC 2010):

> Competency 2:4. All nurses must recognise when people are anxious or in distress and respond effectively, using therapeutic principles to promote their wellbeing, manage personal safety and resolve conflict. They must use effective communication strategies and negotiation techniques to achieve best outcomes, respecting the dignity and human rights of all concerned. They must know when to consult a third party and how to make referrals for advocacy, mediation or arbitration.

Going to theatre

Mr Roberts has chosen to walk to the operating theatre as it is close to the day care unit, and he is escorted by you and an operating department practitioner from the operating theatre area. He informs you that he is a bit worried about his operation, but once he meets the surgeon who is to undertake the surgery and the anaesthetist who he had previously met, he is reassured. He also expresses his thanks to you for staying with him so that you can explain to him what will happen on return to the ward.

The anaesthetist explains that he will be receiving an anaesthetic together with another drug to ensure he does not feel nausea postoperatively, and that he will also receive something to alleviate any postoperative pain. He is having the inguinal hernia repaired using a laparoscope (keyhole surgery) (See Kurzer et al (2007) for an explanation of various techniques).

According to Oakley (2010:39):

> ... the ideal anaesthetic for the day surgery patient should produce very little cardio-respiratory depression, and the induction should be smooth and rapid. The anaesthetic must facilitate the fast turnover of day surgery without pain and postoperative nausea and vomiting, and a rapid return of psychomotor state with minimal hangover effects, allowing for a prompt discharge.

In theatre

You stay with Mr Roberts during the procedure after explaining to the nurse in charge (with your mentor) that you are

Activity

Go to the NHS Choices website for details of a hernia repair:
http://www.nhs.uk/Conditions/ Primaryrepairoffemoralhernia/Pages/ Howisitdonepage.aspx (accessed July 2011).

And see this page for the method of conducting a laparoscopy: http://www. nhs.uk/Conditions/Laparoscopy/ Pages/How-it-is-performed.aspx (accessed July 2011).

See Chapter 7 for details of preparation for undergoing an anaesthetic.

his named nurse and that you are following the total patient care pathway. She is happy for you to stay with him but asks that you put on a sterile gown and gloves and that you learn how to undertake a surgical scrub (see Ch. 8).

Mr Roberts is anaesthetised and the laparoscopic repair of his inguinal hernia is carried out. Although there is a risk of accidental damage to the bowel during this procedure, the surgeon carries out a successful operation and the anaesthetist begins to lighten the anaesthetic in readiness for a short stay in the recovery area (see Ch. 9), although normally patients are returned to the ward straight from the operating theatre (Oakley 2010).

Back on the ward

Once the recovery ward staff and the anaesthetist are satisfied that Mr Roberts has recovered sufficiently from the anaesthetic and that his airway is not compromised, you escort him back to the ward area along with a qualified nurse who has arrived to ensure safety both for the patient and yourself as a student nurse.

Observations for temperature, pulse and respirations (TPR), blood pressure

and any pain experienced by Mr Roberts are carried out. Any postoperative nausea and vomiting will also be managed if required. Although initially nauseated, he does not vomit, and he was given an antiemetic prior to surgery to help him overcome any nausea. As he was admitted in the morning, he should go home in the afternoon. Once the relevant members of the ward staff are happy that he is managing any pain and his observations are normal, he will be encouraged to take oral fluids and some light food, such as toast and a cup of tea. Although he has some discomfort and feels bloated following the laparoscopy (due to carbon dioxide used to inflate the abdomen), he is happy with his progress and care. His wife is contacted and the checklist of criteria for discharge after day surgery is adhered to (see Box 10.3 in Ch. 10). The staff in the unit are satisfied with his postoperative progress, and he has urinated and is tolerating fluids and a light diet.

Going home

His wife arrives to take him home. He is given a discharge letter for his GP and instructions on what, and what not, to do until his follow-up appointment. Any questions he or his wife still have are answered by the nurse who is discharging him from hospital.

He thanks you for staying with him and offers you positive feedback as a service user.

If it is possible and Mr Roberts agrees, following discussion with your mentor, he can complete a service user assessment form to include in your portfolio. This would provide informative feedback and be part of your ongoing record of achievement (NMC 2010).

All patients discharged from hospital after day surgery require follow-up care in the community. A letter is forwarded or given to the patient to take to his GP. A summary of patient advice following discharge is given in Box 11.2. Refer also to Chapter 10 on discharge from hospital.

Box 11.2 Summary of patient advice on discharge

- *How and when to take medication, if any is required.*
- *How to manage wound care, e.g. when to remove any dressings.*
- *When to bathe/shower while any sutures/staples are in place.*
- *When and what exercises can be taken.*
- *When to return to work.*
- *When to start driving following surgery.*
- *Advice about diet and fluids, e.g. to avoid alcohol for 24 hours postoperatively.*
- *Whether a follow-up appointment is necessary in the outpatient clinic.*
- *When any sutures/staples will be removed.*
- *Warnings about nausea and light-headedness that may occur.*
- *What activities may or may not be carried out in the immediate postoperative period, e.g. not to drive a car or operate machinery for 24 hours following discharge.*

(From Oakley 2010:42)

Activity

Reflect on any experiences you have had of caring for patients like Mr Roberts during their stay in the day care unit and write a diary of this experience for your learning portfolio. This experience will make a significant contribution to how you achieve your NMC (2010) Essential Skills and Competencies.

References

Holland, K., Jenkins, J., Solomon, J., Whittam, S., 2008. Applying the Roper, Logan and Tierney model in practice. Churchill Livingstone, Edinburgh.

Kurzer, M., Kark, A., Hussein, T., 2007. Inguinal hernia repair. Journal of Perioperative Practice 17 (7), 318–329.

Nursing and Midwifery Council, 2010. Standards for pre-registration nursing education. NMC, London. Online. Available at: http://standards.nmc-uk. org/PreRegNursing/statutory/ background/Pages/introduction.aspx (accessed September 2011).

Oakley, M., 2010. Day surgery. In: Pudner, R. (Ed.), Nursing the surgical patient, 3rd ed. Baillière Tindall, Edinburgh: 35–44.

Oakley, M., Bratchell, J., 2010. Preoperative assessment. In: Pudner, R. (Ed.), Nursing the surgical patient, 3rd ed. Baillière Tindall, Edinburgh: 3–13.

Pudner, R., 2010. Nursing the surgical patient, 3rd ed. Baillière Tindall, Edinburgh.

Waugh, A., Grant, A., 2010. Ross and Wilson anatomy and physiology in health and illness, 11th ed. Churchill Livingstone, Edinburgh.

Websites

NICE laparoscopic inguinal hernia repair guidelines: http://www.nice.org.uk/ nicemedia/pdf/TA083guidance.pdf (accessed December 2011).

NICE hernia – laparoscopic surgery review: http://guidance.nice.org.uk/TA83 (accessed December 2011).

12

Case study 2: caring for a patient in a general surgical ward

CHAPTER AIMS

- To enable you to reflect on prior learning from other chapters
- To explore in more detail through one specific case study the kind of surgical interventions you may come across in caring for patients in a general surgical ward
- To focus on the total care of a patient who may be admitted onto a general surgical ward, from pre-admission to discharge home and care in the community
- To enable you to identify learning opportunities as well as meeting your practice learning outcomes

occur. In this chapter, we explore the care of a patient who has had a medical diagnosis of cancer of the bowel, identified following the NHS over-60s bowel screening initiative (NHS Bowel Cancer Screening Programme 2009). It is beyond the scope of this book to cover everything with regards to caring for someone after major abdominal surgery. It is advisable, therefore, that you supplement the information in this chapter with that in other chapters plus relevant further reading.

As with the other case studies, it is important to consider them as 'insights' into possible learning experiences in practice placements, where you may meet the patient at any stage in that journey. It is important to learn about the whole of a patient's journey and experience in order to be able to help them at the stage at which you meet them.

Introduction

Patients admitted to a general surgical ward have a short-term stay of a few days or a longer stay of a week or more, depending on the type of surgery and whether any perioperative complications

Introduction to patient and clinical problem

Mrs Nadira Ahmad is a 62-year-old woman who responded to the over-60s bowel screening initiative after seeing an advert for it at her local hospital. A test kit was sent to her and she found this helpful as it meant she could do it in the privacy of her own home, even though she still found it embarrassing. She had been concerned as she had experienced some rectal bleeding and had not told anyone, but she knew from information in her GP centre that 'something was not right' – the poster in the hospital had triggered further inquiry when she realised she could do something without alerting too many people, especially her family. She had been experiencing a change in her normal bowel movements and some discomfort on the right side of her abdomen which she had put down to ingesting the wrong kind of food and 'wind'. She had also been very tired which she had put down to her age.

Two weeks later, Nadira Ahmad receives a letter telling her that she needs to contact the screening service to make an appointment to see a specialist nurse. She is informed that her GP has been sent a letter as well explaining why she needs to contact the nurse. If she prefers, she may go to her GP who knows her and her family as well as her health history.

She is now very concerned. She has asked her daughter, who she eventually confided in, to look for any information on the Internet, and a link from the cancer screening programme site led them to video information about the bowel, polyps and possible investigation of colonoscopy for cancer. This is in her own language of Urdu, which helps her: http://www.remedica.com/bowel/default.aspx (accessed December 2011).

Activity

In order to help patients such as Nadira Ahmad, you need to understand the physiology of the gastrointestinal tract as well as the nature of polyps and why they can turn cancerous.

If you are in a day surgery unit or an outpatient department where colonoscopies are carried out, you will need to communicate effectively with patients and be mindful of different cultural and religious backgrounds as well as your own communication skills.

View the online explanation for the physician about polyps and colonoscopies on the same site: http://www.remedica.com/bowel/default.aspx (accessed December 2011).

Activity

Access the NHS Cancer Screening site and read the information about the initiative and the process prior to the patient receiving the screening test kit. See the link to the information and the kit instructions. A short animated film can also be found there as well as instructions in different languages: http://www.cancerscreening.nhs.uk/bowel/ (accessed December 2011).

Information for GPs is also available for this initiative as they are not directly involved in the delivery of the programme: http://www.cancerscreening.nhs.uk/bowel/ipc-pack.html (accessed December 2011).

See Box 12.1 for an explanation of what the NHS screening site states about colonoscopy for service users and the general public.

Activity

Read the definition in Box 12.1 and compose a more detailed explanation in order to teach another student what happens in a colonoscopy. What would you say differently? For example, would you use the term 'back passage' in your explanation or would the word 'rectum' be more appropriate?

Do not forget how important words are. In some languages, direct translation is not possible, so other non-verbal explanations or illustrations might be required. Again, this is a skill that is transferrable to other situations.

Box 12.1 What is a colonoscopy?

A colonoscopy is an investigation that involves looking directly at the lining of the large bowel. A thin flexible tube with a tiny camera attached (a colonoscope) is passed into the back passage and guided around the bowel. If polyps are found, most can be removed painlessly using a wire tube passed down the colonoscope tube.

(From NHS Bowel Cancer Screening Programme 2009:8)

There are references to physiology textbooks throughout this book and you may have one that you have a personal preference for. To help patients like Nadira Ahmad, it is important that you are fully prepared to answer any questions you feel confident to answer within your sphere of knowledge and responsibility. Being knowledgeable about how the bowel works and what happens in a colonoscopy is essential both pre- and postoperatively should she require major surgery.

Communicating with her in a culturally appropriate way is also very important, as it is with all patients.

Attending for a colonoscopy

After contacting the specialist nurse at the local screening centre, Nadira Ahmad arranges an appointment and her daughter accompanies her. Here is what happens at the clinic.

Nurse-led clinic

This is a 45 minute consultation to allow you to discuss with the Specialist Screening Practitioner any concerns you may have about your results. The Nurse will explain about the next investigation which is called colonoscopy.

She will assess your health to see whether you are suitable to have the next investigation. A Health Questionnaire will be completed so it is important to bring information with you about the tablets you take.

The Nurse will also explain about the diet you need to follow three days before colonoscopy and the bowel preparation you need to take 24 hours before your investigation.

(From http://www.mccn.nhs.uk/patients/tests/screening/bowel-screening-process.php (accessed December 2011)).

Activity

During your clinical placement in either surgical nursing or community nursing, organising an insight day or a 2–3-day spoke placement is very helpful for understanding the patient experience,

Continued

communication skills and the role of the nurse in this type of new screening service. It is also important for understanding health policy such as that which has influenced the introduction of this screening programme across the UK.

Read the article by Coutts (2010) (see References) for the main report explaining the rationale for the initiation of the bowel screening programme.

In addition there is a report on Ethnicity and Uptake of Bowel Cancer Screening Pilot study (NHS 2003) which will help you consider some of the experiences of Nadira Ahmad. Read also the systematic review of the evidence of the uptake of cancer screening services internationally.

http://www.cancerscreening.nhs.uk/bowel/ethnicity-finalreport.pdf (accessed December 2011).

Nadira Ahmad agrees to attend for a colonoscopy following the meeting with the nurse and her daughter agrees to share this with the rest of the family – her two brothers and their wives. Her husband died 2 years previously at age 68 from lung cancer, so she was very aware of what might happen if she had not responded to her concerns.

An appointment is made for the following week's colonoscopy clinic and instructions given to her regarding bowel preparation and her diet in the week before the investigation.

The colonoscopy

Re-visit the online information on this procedure at http://www.remedica.com/bowel/default.aspx (accessed December 2011).

Colonoscopies are normally carried out in a specialised endoscopy unit. This is somewhere you and your mentor could discuss as a possible insight visit or you may actually have a longer placement in a unit like this. In any case,

you will gain excellent learning opportunities in patient care, including sedation and post-procedure care, communication skills and multidisciplinary team working.

Following the procedure, Nadira Ahmad and her daughter are asked to speak to the doctor, which obviously upsets them. He explains that he has found an unusual mass which he has diagnosed as cancer of the bowel. He also explains that early detection of bowel cancer normally results in a 90% chance of it being treated successfully.

He discusses with her the main outcome of this finding – the necessity for surgical intervention – and tells her she will need to come for surgery as soon as possible. The nurse then advises her that she will receive a letter inviting her to come to the pre-assessment clinic in the next few days, when more detailed information can be discussed.

Bowel cancer can be found anywhere in the large bowel (see Fig. 12.1).

Surgery possibilities

Nadira Ahmad's tumour was located in the right ascending colon of the large bowel, and there did not appear to be any lymphatic involvement. She was advised that the surgery would probably be a right hemicolectomy – removing the tumour from the ascending colon, the part of the bowel ending in the caecum. In this procedure, a section of the large intestine is removed, including the normal bowel on either side of the diseased part, and the remainder is attached to the lower end of the small intestine (called an anastomosis), usually with stitches or by stapling them together. There would also be external clips or stitches on the abdominal wound which will need to be removed 7–12 days postoperatively (this will likely take place in the community but it depends on her postoperative recovery). She does not require a permanent colostomy/stoma.

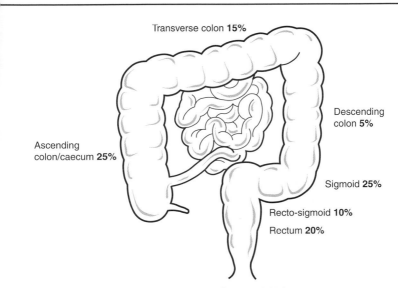

Fig 12.1 Common sites of herniation (Waugh and Grant 2010:321)

It is possible that Nadira Ahmad will stay in hospital from 7 to 10 days after surgery. She is given information from the hospital about the surgery and postoperative care. She is also advised that as she will have major abdominal surgery, she needs to consider postoperative care once she is discharged home from hospital (see Ch. 10). She is given an urgent appointment to attend the pre-admission assessment clinic at the hospital.

Pre-admission assessment

Nadira Ahmad attends the pre-assessment clinic a week prior to admission for her surgery. The clinic she attends is a nurse-led clinic where the nurses organise a chest X-ray, an electrocardiograph (ECG) and blood tests, as well as taking blood pressure measurements. These were determined to be normal for her age.

Given the nature of the surgery, she is also informed of any special requirements with regards to eating, drinking and eliminating, to prepare herself and her bowel for surgery (such as a special diet in the days before surgery and an enema to ensure the bowel is empty, etc. – see Box 12.2) (Hibberts 2010).

A very important task undertaken by the anaesthetist and her doctor is obtaining informed consent (see Ch. 6). They must ensure that she completely understands the intended surgery and that, if necessary, they are allowed to make other decisions based on what they find during the surgery itself.

Her daughter is also involved at this stage.

⚙ Activity

Re-read Chapter 5 on pre-admission to hospital and undertake a plan of care for Nadira Ahmad from your experiences and/or using the information in that chapter.

Box 12.2 Specific issues related to preoperative bowel preparation (if required)

- *Potential risk of infection if bowel not adequately cleansed.*
- *Operation cancelled due to inadequate preparation.*
- *Potential loss of fluid and electrolytes due to physical preparation/dehydration from the cleansing solutions.*
- *Potential risk of abdominal pain caused by physical preparation.*
- *Specific objective will be to ensure that the bowel is clean prior to surgery and to minimise the side effects of vomiting and abdominal pain.*

Nursing intervention and rationale

- *Ensure the physical cleansing preparation procedure is correctly carried out and instructions for any laxatives or irrigation are carefully followed and monitored. The result of the preparation should be fully documented, and any difficulty in carrying out the procedure should be reported to the surgeon who is performing the surgery.*
- *All fluid loss associated with diarrhoea and vomiting should be recorded on appropriate documentation, thereby ensuring that fluid and electrolytes can be replaced by intravenous infusion. Antiemetics may be used to relieve excessive nausea and vomiting.*
- *Identify characteristics of the abdominal pain, duration and intensity, and provide appropriate analgesics, ensuring effectiveness is evaluated. Any associated discomfort through diarrhoea is relieved by ensuring the anal area is clean and dry following any bowel action and by providing anaesthetic creams and protective barrier creams.*

(From Hibberts 2010:341)

Preoperative care

Nadira Ahmad is admitted to hospital (where you are undertaking a clinical placement) a week later. She has followed the regime set out for her prior to admission and has been admitted the day before her surgery so she can become familiar with the ward and staff and meet one of the hospital interpreters who may be required to help her understand explanations of procedures or aspects of care, if necessary (see Holland & Hogg (2010) for discussion of the interpreter role).

Your mentor is her named nurse and has asked you to become her co-named nurse during the patient's stay in hospital.

Activity

If Nadira Ahmad was your patient, agree with your mentor how you can experience all aspects of her care in hospital, and subsequently visit her in the community on her discharge home. You and your mentor would be able to liaise with the community team as she lives close to the hospital.

Work out one **SMART** (**S**pecific, **M**easurable, **A**ttainable, **R**elevant and **T**imely) goal to meet your learning needs with regards to a patient undergoing major abdominal surgery.

Note: a SMART Goal is one that is:

S = Specific (clear and well defined);

M = Measurable (can see how much time you are going to take to do it); A = Attainable (Achievable - possible to achieve them in the time set); R = Relevant (need to be relevant to the placement experience and your learning needs) and T = Time-bound (have a deadline by the time you need to complete it).

Theatre and recovery

Nadira Ahmad is escorted to the anaesthetic room by yourself and the operating theatre practitioner who has been sent to bring her to the anaesthetic room.

Re-visit Chapter 7 to see what happens in the anaesthetic room.

You tell Nadira Ahmad that you will stay with her during the whole of the surgery, including the operation and the recovery room time. She is obviously much relieved by this and keeps hold of your hand until the anaesthesia has begun to work and she is wheeled into the operating theatre.

Activity

Re-visit theatre practice and the gowning up process. You may get an opportunity to see the surgeon performing the surgery which is an excellent opportunity to link the theory of anatomy and physiology of the bowel. It will also allow you to explain to Nadira Ahmad postoperatively why she may experience symptoms such as pain and why she can't eat immediately afterwards.

Postoperative care

Nadira Ahmad returns to the ward with you accompanying her, following a good recovery in theatre. Back on the ward, she is given postoperative analgesia and an antiemetic. She is commenced on a pain pump. You explain to her, through the interpreter as her daughter has gone home to put her children to bed, how this works and how she can use it.

She is receiving intravenous fluids to replace fluid and electrolytes lost in theatre, and has already had 2 units of blood in the recovery room to replace some blood loss.

You commence observations according to the instructions of the anaesthetist and these are found to be within normal limits for her and for the postoperative period following major surgery. She is recovering well. She is given hourly mouth care as she is not drinking and her mouth, to begin with, is very dry.

Activity

Watch the videos identified in previous chapters on all aspects of postoperative care, such as:

http://www.cetl.org.uk/learning/tutorials.html (accessed December 2011).

Another website with additional clinical skills resources and material on observations, injection giving and other skills is:

http://www.oup.com/uk/orc/bin/9780199237838/01student/video/ (accessed December 2011).

Nadira Ahmad has returned from surgery with a catheter in place due to events during the operation and the surgeon has given instructions that it should be removed after 48 hours.

She keeps asking for a drink of water but you explain that, at the moment, she is unable to have this. You make sure her mouth is cared for to stimulate saliva and make her mouth feel refreshed.

Bowel sounds are heard after 48 hours and she passes flatus (wind) which means that she can commence fluids and, once tolerated, she will be started on an appropriate diet postoperatively and according to her cultural needs. Her catheter is removed and although she initially finds it difficult to pass urine, she eventually manages to do so.

She does not experience a paralytic ileus due to the handling of the bowel in surgery (see Hibberts 2010:341), and is making a very good postoperative recovery.

Her wound has a drain which is checked regularly and managed according to the amount of drainage along with observation of the fluid exudate. No infection is noted and the drain is removed after 4 days, when drainage is less that 50 ml per day (Endacott et al 2009: 116–123).

◎ Activity

Plan Nadira Ahmad's care after the first 48 hours. Include aspects of sexuality and changing body image, pain management, elimination, managing her diet, postoperatively following major abdominal surgery. In addition wound management and principles of wound care (see Endacott et al 2009: 114–123).

Key aspects can be found in Sections 1 and 2 but you may need to read further about the specific care of a patient who has had a hemicolectomy for bowel cancer. It is also important to consider all her care in relation to her cultural needs (see Holland et al 2008).

Discharge home from hospital

Because of Nadira Ahmad's good postoperative recovery and having someone to help her at home, she is discharged home 7 days after surgery.

She is tolerating a light diet, passing water and has had two bowel movements

resulting in soft stools after beginning to eat and commencing free fluids.

Some of her sutures (interrupted) are removed before she is discharged home, but your mentor has decided that at least three of them need to remain for at least another 2 days. They will require removal after her discharge home by the district/community nurse.

Instructions about her postoperative recovery and follow-up nursing treatments are given to Nadira Ahmad and also sent to her GP and the district nurse.

◎ Activity

Undertake a plan of discharge from hospital for Nadira Ahmad and then one for a patient of your choice following major surgery as part of your assessment of competency in nursing practice and decision making (Nursing and Midwifery Council 2010).

Recovery from surgery at home

Once home, Nadira Ahmad is apprehensive about her wound and diet, and wants to know whether her cancer has gone. She has an appointment in the outpatient clinic in 6 weeks' time but tries to allay some of her concerns by asking her daughter to phone the health centre and make an appointment to see her GP. The district nurse has already visited, and as Nadira Ahmad is visiting her GP in 2 days time, she organises to take her sutures out in the health centre at the same time. She also organises for her to see the specialist nurse who she saw at the beginning of her surgical journey in order to answer more specific questions related to her bowel cancer and future monitoring of her susceptibility to the disease.

Summary

This case history is a brief introduction to the care of a patient who has undergone major surgery. By following a patient's journey in this way, you can maximise your learning by thinking of this as a placement learning pathway. You might discuss with your mentor the possibility of doing the same with a patient you are caring for in your surgical placement.

References

Coutts, A., 2010. The bowel cancer screening programme: Understanding the rationale. Gastrointestinal Nursing 8 (3), 38–41.

Endacott, R., Jevon, P., Cooper, S., 2009. Clinical nursing skills: core and advanced. Oxford University Press, Oxford.

Hibberts, F., 2010. Patients requiring colorectal and anal surgery. In: Pudner, R. (Ed.), Nursing the surgical patient. Baillière Tindall, Edinburgh: 325–348.

Holland, K., Hogg, C., 2010. Cultural awareness in nursing and healthcare, 2nd ed. Arnold, London.

Holland, K., Jenkins, J., Solomon, J., Whittam, S., 2008. Applying the Roper, Logan and Tierney model in practice. Churchill Livingstone, Edinburgh.

NHS Bowel Cancer Screening Programme, 2009. Online. Available at: http://www.cancerscreening.nhs.uk/bowel/ (accessed December 2011).

Nursing and Midwifery Council, 2010. Standards for pre-registration nursing education. NMC, London. Online. Available at: http://standards.nmc-uk.org/PreRegNursing/statutory/background/Pages/introduction.aspx (accessed September 2011).

Further reading

Black, P., 2009. Cultural and religious beliefs in stoma care nursing. British Journal of Nursing 18 (13), 790–793.

Narayanasamy, A., 2003. Transcultural nursing: how do nurses respond to cultural needs? British Journal of Nursing 12 (3), 185–194.

Websites

NHS Choices website. Stories of life experiences of having been diagnosed or treated with bowel cancer: http://www.nhs.uk/Conditions/Cancer-of-the-colon-rectum-or-bowel/Pages/Lindas-story.aspx (accessed December 2011).

Merseyside and Cheshire NHS Cancer Network. Nurse led screening service: http://www.mccn.nhs.uk/patients/tests/screening/bowel-screening-process.php (accessed August 2011).

13 Case study 3: caring for a patient requiring emergency surgery

CHAPTER AIMS

- To enable you to reflect on prior learning from other chapters
- To explore in more detail through one specific case study the kind of surgical interventions you may come across in an emergency care situation
- To focus on the total care of a patient who may be admitted to an orthopaedic ward from an accident and emergency unit for surgery, from admission to discharge home and care in the community
- To enable you to identify learning opportunities as well as meeting your practice learning outcomes

Introduction

Some patients you will care for during your clinical placement will have been admitted to hospital via the emergency services, usually through the accident and emergency (A&E) department or similar named units. This can be a traumatic experience not only for the patient but also for their families, carers, friends and sometimes even the nursing staff working in the department. This chapter focuses on a patient journey from the A&E department to the orthopaedic ward where you are undertaking your clinical placement experience.

 Activity

Re-visit Section 1, in particular the key principles, placement learning opportunities and terminology used in clinical placements identified as surgical.

Introduction to patient and clinical problem

Mrs Elsie Waters is an 80-year-old woman who lives on her own in a small bungalow that has been adapted to her needs. Her son and his family live close by and he or his wife call every day to see if she needs anything. He has also ensured she has a mobile phone in case she requires help and she uses it to call with any shopping or other needs.

On this particular day, her son let himself into the house, calling to his mother that he had arrived and asking where she was. Not getting any reply, he became worried and started to search the bungalow. He heard a weak call for help and found his mother on the floor of the bedroom with the mobile phone some distance away. It was clear she had fallen for some reason and articles from the bedside table were all over the floor. She was weak but was able to tell her son that her right hip hurt and she was unable to move that leg.

He immediately called an ambulance and placed a pillow underneath his mother's head but did not move her until they arrived. Within 10 minutes, the paramedic team arrived, assessed the situation and made a provisional diagnosis of a fractured neck of femur. They ensured a safe transfer from the floor onto a stretcher and informed her and her son that they would be taking her to the hospital. Her son told them he would sort out some clothes and other things for her, as it was clear she would be required to stay in hospital, and that he would follow them. He phoned his wife at work to let her know about his mother and

that he would be going to the hospital with his mother and that he would phone back once she had been seen by the doctor in the A&E department.

Falls in the elderly population

Being mobile is very important to an older person like Mrs Waters and, like her, many live independent lives. However, Hindle (2011) states that, according to Help the Aged data, falls in the elderly 'represent over half of hospital admissions for accidental injury – particularly hip fracture' (Help the Aged 2005).

Activity

Access the Help the Aged website (now merged with others and known as Age UK) and consider the issues involved in falls and the elderly so that you are better able to answer any questions that Mrs Waters and her relatives might ask. There is a campaign to reduce the number of falls in older people.

http://www.ageuk.org.uk/get-involved/campaign/falls/ (accessed December 2011).

There is also a range of other useful information and reports which will support your developing knowledge base of caring for elderly people in clinical placements.

Activity

If your placement is in the orthopaedic ward discuss with your mentor the possibility of spending some time in the A&E department to see what happens when a patient with trauma of some kind arrives via ambulance, what the role of the nurse is and the treatment and care that patients like Mrs Waters would experience. Set yourself a **SMART** (**S**pecific, **M**easurable, **A**ttainable, **R**elevant and **T**imely) goal with your personal tutor and mentor to achieve a learning outcome in relation to emergency care prior to surgery.

Consider also the risk factors involving older people and falls in their own homes.

Admission to hospital

When Mrs Waters arrives at the A&E department, she is experiencing a great deal of pain in her right hip and side, she has a cut on her head (which is thought to have happened when she fell and hit her head on the corner of her bedside table), her pulse rate is raised and she is very pale. She is also worried about her cat and who is going to look after him. Her son arrives and reassures her about this latter concern.

 Activity

Revise the anatomy and physiology of the femur and hip joint. Consider what part of the femur could be fractured and look up the types of surgery Mrs Waters might have.

Paper to read prior to placement:

Malik, A.A., Kell, P., Khan, W.S., et al., 2009. Surgical management of fractured neck of femur. Journal of Perioperative Practice 19(3), 100–104.

This paper shows many different X-rays of fractures and their surgical treatment, such as pinning and plating and internal screw insertion.

Immediate care in the A&E department

The Scottish Intercollegiate Guidelines Network (SIGN) guidance (SIGN 2002) would be used to guide the perioperative period of care for Mrs Waters, including the immediate management in the A&E department. The guidelines (section 4) recommend early assessment and recording of the following, either in A&E or if admitted first prior to surgery on the ward (SIGN 2002):

- *Pressure sore risk.*
- *Hydration and nutrition.*
- *Fluid balance.*
- *Pain.*

- *Core body temperature using a low reading thermometer.*
- *Continence.*
- *Co-existing medical problems.*
- *Mental state.*
- *Previous mobility.*
- *Previous functional ability.*
- *Social circumstances, including whether the patient has a carer (SIGN 2009).*

They also suggest there should be immediate steps taken to prevent the development of pressure sores and that those at high risk of developing pressure sores should be assessed using appropriate assessment tools. They recommend that any patient admitted to A&E with a suspected hip fracture should also be managed as detailed in Box 13.1.

> **Box 13.1** Immediate management of a patient with suspected hip fracture
>
> - Use soft surfaces to protect the heel and sacrum from pressure damage.
> - Keep the patient warm.
> - Administer adequate pain relief to allow for regular comfortable change of patient position.
> - Instigate early radiology.
> - Measure and correct any fluid and electrolyte abnormalities.

The triage nurse assesses Mrs Waters as someone who requires to be seen immediately by the doctor and who requires pain relief and an X-ray in order to make a diagnosis and also to make her more comfortable. Pain relief is ordered by the doctor and given by the staff nurse looking after Mrs Waters, prior to her being moved from the trolley to the X-ray table. The nurse accompanies her to the radiography unit which is next to the A&E department so that patients can easily be transported and returned.

Activity

Read up on the main types of analgesia that could be given to Mrs Waters and discuss them with your mentor. If you are in an orthopaedic ward for your placement, ask to spend time in the A&E department as part of your ongoing placement learning experience and learning agreement for this placement.

Paper to read prior to placement:

Layzell, M., 2009 Exploring pain management in older people with hip fracture. Nursing Times 105(2), 20–23.

This article offers a comprehensive review of pain management in older people with hip fractures.

Return from X-ray

Mrs Waters returns from X-ray and a diagnosis of a fracture of the femoral neck or an intracapsular fracture is made. This type of fracture involves an injury whereby the 'ball' or femoral head is broken off from the main shaft. Treatment will vary according to age, previous health and the condition of the bone and joint itself. Main treatments are either an internal fixation (of the broken off head and the femur shaft) or hemiarthroplasty (part hip replacement of the femoral head into the undamaged socket). Sometimes a total hip replacement of both head and socket may be required. As Mrs Waters is 80 years old, does not suffer from dementia and is normally very mobile, it is decided that a hemiarthroplasty will be undertaken.

 Activity

Access this NHS website, read about hip fractures and watch the short video about hip fractures, their causes and treatment:

http://www.nhs.uk/Conditions/hip-fracture/Pages/introduction.aspx (accessed September 2011).

Going to the operating theatre

Mrs Waters is taken to the orthopaedic ward from the A&E department to become familiar with staff and the surroundings on return from the operating theatre and also to enable the nursing staff on the ward to prepare her for surgery. Due to the timing of her fall, she has not eaten or drunk anything for some time, and an intravenous infusion has already been commenced in the A&E department. Her son has remained with her during admission and this has helped the nursing staff considerably, as she has someone familiar with her who has been able to contribute information regarding his her health and prior mobility.

The surgeon who is to carry out the surgery later that morning is on the ward when she arrives and is able to speak with her and her son. He also obtains consent for the surgery to take place and ensures that the right leg is marked ready for the surgery. She is prepared for theatre by the ward nurses and postoperative care is explained to her.

 Activity

Watch this video focusing on a total hip replacement and identify the multidisciplinary members of the surgical team:

http://www.royalfree.org.uk/default.aspx?sel_left_nav=25&tab_id=868&top_nav_id=1 (accessed December 2011).

Discuss with your personal tutor and/or mentor all the stages of the surgery discussed in this very informative video. Consider the difference in care between the woman in the video and Mrs Waters, who has been admitted as an emergency.

Activity

Read Chapters 6–8 and consider Mrs Waters' care until the end of surgery. Using a recognised care plan and a framework, write a possible care plan for Mrs Waters, identifying potential and actual problems she is like to experience postoperatively.

Immediate postoperative care: first 48 hours

Mrs Waters undergoes a hemiarthroplasty, with a new head of femur inserted. She is taken to the recovery ward for immediate observations and care. See Box 13.2 for the SIGN consensus statement on instructions for discharge from the recovery area, together with essential aspects of patient recovery criteria.

As soon as Mrs Waters meets the criteria for discharge from the recovery area, she is taken back to the ward by a recovery room nurse and a nurse from the ward. (If your mentor is one of these, take the opportunity to request that you go with her to collect the patient so that you can gain an understanding of the handover process in the recovery room, including what the anaesthetist and surgical team have written in relation to her care and treatment during surgery and in the recovery room.)

Box 13.2 Criteria for discharge from the recovery room (as per Scottish Intercollegiate Network Consensus Statement)

The following criteria must be fulfilled before a patient can be discharged from the recovery room:

- The patient is fully conscious, responding to voice or light touch, able to maintain a clear airway and has a normal cough reflex.
- Respiration and oxygen saturation are satisfactory (10–20 breaths per minute and $SpO_2 > 92\%$).
- The cardiovascular system is stable with no unexplained cardiac irregularity or persistent bleeding.
- The patient's pulse and blood pressure should approximate to normal preoperative values or should be at a level commensurate with the planned postoperative care.
- Pain and emesis should be controlled and suitable analgesic and antiemetic regimens should be prescribed.
- Temperature should be within acceptable limits ($> 36°C$).
- Oxygen and fluid therapy should be prescribed when required.

Anaesthetic and surgical staff should record the following in the patient's case notes:

- any anaesthetic, surgical or intraoperative complications
- any specific postoperative instructions concerning possible problems
- any specific treatment or prophylaxis required (e.g. fluids, nutrition, antibiotics, analgesia, antiemetics, thromboprophylaxis).

Activity

Re-visit Chapter 9 and plan Mrs Waters' immediate care on arrival back on the ward. Make a note of key issues to consider in this plan including, for example, that she was admitted originally as an emergency.

Activity

Read Ryan 2008 (see References). Consider your care plan and determine the difference between rehabilitation following a hemiarthroplasty, as Mrs Waters had, and the alternative surgery of an internal fixation with screws and a plate.

Postoperative care after return to the ward until discharge home

Mrs Waters made a good postoperative recovery and does not experience the confusion that many elderly patients experience following orthopaedic surgery. However, she was slightly disorientated during her first 2 nights postoperatively (see Rogers & Gibson's [2002] study of the experiences of nurses caring for elderly patients with acute confusion). She could also have experienced problems such as constipation, e.g. due to lack of mobility, opioid analgesics, different diet, or, if she had a catheter inserted, a urinary tract infection. This is normally avoided if at all possible (SIGN 2002, Guideline 8.6).

The physiotherapist linked to the ward visits Mrs Waters in the first 24 hours postoperatively to introduce herself and to assess her ability to move. She begins rehabilitation with the physiotherapist 48 hours after surgery.

Ryan (2008) identifies some standard protocols for early mobilisation after surgery for a fractured hip. These are listed in Box 13.3.

As mentioned, Mrs Waters did not experience any major post-operative confusion as described by Wong et al (2002:69) but she was disorientated at night and not during the day:

> Delirium or post-operative acute confusion state (ACS) is a transient disorder of cognition and is a significant

Box 13.3 Standard protocols for early mobilisation after surgery for a fractured hip (Ryan 2008)

First postoperative day

- *Hip movement precautions (after replacement of the femoral head, some movements are prohibited, e.g. flexion beyond 90°, adduction past the midline and internal rotation).*
- *Active range of movement for other limbs.*
- *Isometric exercises of the affected limb to strengthen quadriceps and gluteal muscles.*

Second postoperative day

- *Observe hip precautions.*
- *Practice transfers and mobility in bed.*
- *Assisted standing while observing weight-bearing restrictions.*

Third postoperative day onwards

- *Walk short distances using walking aid.*
- *Observe weight-bearing restrictions.*

> problem among elderly surgical patients. The incidence of acute confusion varies widely. In an extensive review of the literature Foreman (1993) concluded that acute confusion among elderly typically occurred between 24 hours and 6 days after admission to an acute setting.

They also noted that *'the incidence of post-operative confusion is greater in orthopaedic than in general surgery'* (Wong, 2002:69).

Discharge from hospital and rehabilitation following a fractured femur

Mrs Waters' postoperative recovery was good and her prior good health was of benefit in this. Her son and daughter-in-law came to the ward to discuss with the surgeon and the nursing staff what the best rehabilitation process would be for her, and she was actively involved in this discussion process. This was very important for her psychologically as well as recognising her individual views in decision making.

It was agreed that she would live with her family for the first 6 weeks post-discharge until her follow-up appointment at the orthopaedic clinic, then they would discuss whether she could go back home to live on her own again.

Mrs Waters thought this was the best choice for her.

She was therefore discharged home with her postoperative instructions, including the importance of not dislocating the new head of femur.

An example of patient information discharge advice is given in Box 13.4.

Activity

With your mentor, design a pathway of learning experience that meets your Nursing and Midwifery Council learning outcomes and also your own personal goals of caring for patients undergoing orthopaedic surgery. Plan insight learning days with a number of members of the multidisciplinary team or a longer spoke placement either in the orthopaedic operating theatre or following a patient such as Mrs Waters on her discharge home from hospital by liaising with the community nurses responsible for her care.

Box 13.4 Patient Information Discharge Advice

Swelling

It is not uncommon to have swollen ankles for at least 3 months following your surgery. You are advised to rest in bed for 1–2 hours in the afternoon to help reduce the swelling.

If your calf becomes swollen and tense to the touch it may be a sign that you have developed a DVT. It is important that you contact your GP urgently or attend the Accident & Emergency Department for further advice and treatment.

Painkillers

Only take the tablets you were given on discharge. As the pain eases, these should gradually be reduced. If you require any help or information regarding your medication on discharge, please contact your GP.

Stitches/clips

These will be removed 14 days after the operation by either your practice nurse or district nurse, or if you remain in hospital by a nurse on the ward.

(From Ashford and St Peter's Hospitals NHS Foundation Trust 2011)

Activity

Do continue with your exercise regime as taught to you by your physiotherapist, and gradually increase the number of times you repeat each exercise as soon as you feel comfortable to do so.

Do go for short walks regularly. Try to slowly increase the amount you are doing each day. The amount you do will not damage your hip but might tire you out at first

Summary

Being admitted as an emergency has a major impact on what happens to patients on admission to hospital and any subsequent postoperative care pathways.

In this brief overview of one such patient, you can begin to understand the kind of care patients such as Mrs Waters experience. Not all patients have swift recoveries when they are 80 years old. During your clinical placement experience, it is important for you to be able to manage the care of older patients in any context. Due to the increasing ageing population, there will be many more elderly patients requiring acute or long-term care.

References

Ashford and St Peter's Hospitals NHS Foundation Trust, 2011. Fractured neck of femur: trauma and orthopaedics. Online. Available at: http://www. ashfordstpeters.nhs.uk/attachments/ 170_Fractured%20Neck%20of% 20Femur.pdf (accessed December 2011).

Hindle, A., 2011. Mobility and falls. In: Hindle, A., Coates, A. (Eds.), Nursing care of older people. Oxford University Press, Oxford.

Layzell, M., 2009. Exploring pain management in older people with hip fracture. Nursing Times 105 (2), 20–23. Online. Available at: http://www. nursingtimes.net/nursing-practice-clinical-research/exploring-pain-management-in-older-people-with-hip-fracture/1970471.article (accessed December 2011).

Malik, A.A., Kell, P., Khan, W.S., et al., 2009. Surgical management of fractured neck of femur. Journal of Perioperative Practice 19 (3), 100–104.

Rogers, A.C., Gibson, C.H., 2002. Experiences of orthopaedic nurses caring for elderly patients with acute confusion. Journal of Orthopaedic Nursing 6, 9–17.

Ryan, J., 2008. Mobilising. In: Holland, K., Jenkins, J., Solomon, J., Whittam, S. (Eds.), Applying the Roper, Logan and Tierney model in practice. Churchill Livingstone, Edinburgh: 357–363.

Scottish Intercollegiate Guidelines Network, 2009. Management of hip fracture in older people: a national clinical guideline. Online. Available at: http:// www.sign.ac.uk/pdf/sign111.pdf (accessed August 2011).

Wong, J., Wong, S., Brooks, E., 2002. A study of hospital recovery pattern of acutely confused older patients following hip surgery. Journal of Orthopaedic Nursing 6, 68–78.

Further reading

Healee, D.J., McCallin, A., Jones, M., 2010. Older adults' recovery from hip fracture: a literature review. International Journal of Orthopaedic and Trauma Nursing 15, 18–28.

Hindle, A., Coates, A., 2011. Nursing care of older people. Oxford University Press, Oxford.

Redfern, S.J., Ross, F.M., 2006. Nursing older people. Churchill Livingstone, Edinburgh.

Robinson, T.N., Eisman, B., 2008. Postoperative delirium in the elderly: diagnosis and management. Clinical Interventions in Aging 3 (2), 351–355. Online. Available at: http://ukpmc.ac.uk/articles/PMC2546478 (accessed September 2011).

Websites

The Scottish Intercollegiate Guidelines Network: management of hip fracture in older people: a national clinical guideline: http://www.sign.ac.uk/pdf/sign111.pdf (accessed August 2011). This website offers access to the full report, together with a range of other information which will help you to understand the principles of caring perioperatively for older people following a hip fracture as well as the surgical management. The report is evidence based.

Ashford and St Peter's Hospitals NHS Foundation Trust: fractured neck of femur – trauma and orthopaedics: http://www.ashfordstpeters.nhs.uk/attachments/170_Fractured%20Neck%20of%20Femur.pdf (accessed September 2011). This links to a patient information booklet given to patients and their relatives to offer an explanation of what has happened to the patient and their treatment and aftercare. It can be obtained in a range of different languages, and includes pictures of the nature of the fracture as well as discharge advice.

Section 4. Consolidating learning

In this section, we re-visit your learning in the other sections and help you reflect on your experiences of learning within a surgical placement.

Examples of potential seminar/revision questions you may encounter with regards to caring for a patient undergoing surgery are considered, together with possible responses in relation to the content found in this book and elsewhere.

It is important also to refer to the Nursing and Midwifery Council standards and domain competencies that you will be achieving in the placement and how your learning in practice can help you, in collaboration with your mentor and others, to gain new skills and consolidate others.

14

What have I learnt in a surgical nursing placement?

CHAPTER AIMS

- To reflect on learning experience in a surgical nursing placement
- To establish what knowledge and skills you have gained during the placement
- To consider how what you have learnt in your surgical nursing placement can be utilised in a range of other placements and in various fields of practice
- To identify the experiences your mentor will use to establish whether you have met your learning goals and/ or competences for the placement

Introduction

Reflecting on your learning is an essential skill to establish early on in your programme of study, to discus with your personal tutor at university and with your mentor in practice. During your time on placement, you will be assessed in accordance with your programme requirements and, most importantly, the Nursing and Midwifery Council (NMC)

standards in the four domains and their generic and field-specific competencies.

This chapter explores the above aims through a range of exercises, references to other chapters and new learning experiences. To begin with, we can re-visit what reflection means and how you do this, in particular reflection on being a student nurse, reflection in the practice of actually 'doing' nursing and what goals you now need to set for the future.

Reflection

Most of you will have come across the term 'reflection' in your programme of study, but what does it mean in the context of learning in clinical practice? How important is it to your learning to become a nurse? We consider these two questions in the context of undertaking any placement experience and also a surgical one.

At the beginning of your programme of study, you will have been given a practical assessment document to be used by yourself, your mentor and personal tutor to assess, record and discuss your learning in practice to meet the requirements of your course and, most importantly, to meet the requirements of the NMC. Along with this document will be some kind of personal portfolio and personal and professional development documentation in which to document your learning experiences throughout your journey to becoming a qualified nurse. You will be expected to continue this practice following successful registration as a qualified nurse, as maintaining your professional development is an NMC requirement to remain a registered nurse, as well as being part of your annual appraisal requirement by your employer if you work in the NHS.

Timmins (2008:1) offers the following definition of what a portfolio is:

*A portfolio is a collection and cohesive account of **work-based learning** that contains relevant **evidence from practice** and **critical reflection on this evidence.** Its primary purpose is to display achievement of **your learning and knowledge development.** Most commonly the portfolio is a hand-held document, such as a ring binder, that you, as a student, carry with you to prepare and complete while you are actually gaining your practical clinical experience within the clinical practice environment; it can also be in electronic format.*

The key words, highlighted in bold, link to the idea of learning from your experiences in clinical placement (workplace learning), evidencing this in some way as written work but, most importantly, reflecting on what you have written about your learning through analysing the experience rather than just describing it. Describing your experiences and what you have learnt from them are both important, but considering them in relation to previous experiences and/or theoretical knowledge can help you to understand what took place or what you felt during the experiences.

It is beyond the scope of this book to discuss reflection and reflective practice in full, but you will find specific texts and articles, such as Timmins (2008) and Hart (2010), to help you at the end of the chapter.

Your portfolio will contain a range of important documents that you are required to have in order to become a nurse registered with the NMC as well as evidence of your personal and professional growth over the course of your programme of study.

What then is reflection? Schon (1983) wrote that there are two types of reflection in relation to clinical practice learning: reflection-in-action and reflection-on-action. The latter is the one we focus on in this chapter but it is also important to consider reflection-in-action as well. Consider the definition of reflection offered by Price and Harrington (2010:25):

... a process whereby experience is examined in ways that give meaning to interaction. We might examine the experience in real time or in retrospect. Because experience engages the emotions as well as reasoning, reflection needs to take account of the feelings engendered within an interaction and to allow that perceptions (how we interpret matters) may sometimes prove erroneous. While reflection is most closely associated with human interactions and especially clinical events, it is not limited to these. We may, for instance, reflect upon the written accounts of experiences, such as those shared by dying patients. Reflection may be used in the service of different nursing goals – those that are designed to tell us something about how we think, what we value and with regard to ways in which practice could be improved.

Reflection, then, involves thinking about what you have done, taking the activity 'out of the box' and looking at it both in terms of how you felt about it when looking at it and actually experiencing or doing it. This is reflection-on-action, the one which you will be asked to write about if doing this for an assignment, to critically review it in terms of evidence, i.e. supporting the rationale for why you did what you did through theoretical concepts or supporting research.

For example, imagine you wrote the following as part of your reflection on an experience with a patient who was going to theatre: *'I asked the patient whether she had any concerns about going to the operating theatre. She wanted to know what would happen in the theatre and so I explained to her the procedure that would be carried out. She seemed relieved to know that it was perfectly normal to feel afraid that she wouldn't wake up'*. We know from previous Chapters the importance of talking to patients and reassuring them before surgery, and the importance of explaining what will happen, for example we would add to the above reflection in the following way to demonstrate critical reflection or reflection based on evidence.

Critical reflection: evidence based

'. . . She wanted to know what would happen in the theatre and so I explained to her the procedure that would be carried out.'

Miller and Webb (2010:59) refer to this as 'attending' to the patient, whereby *'active listening and attending rely on being able to communicate to the other person that we are listening, understanding, remembering, and even interested in what they are communicating.'*

Examining the reflection in 'real time' is actually harder to contemplate, as it is reflection-*in*-action, not actually visible to others nor easily expressed, and refers to looking at what you are doing as it actually happens. What you might be reflecting - *in*-action on may well involve personal feelings of your own or something related specifically to the patient or the situation you have not dealt with before. Imagine a scenario where someone on your ward is having a cardiac arrest. You have never seen one before and only know the key steps to take when it happens, such as calling for help, phoning the right number for the cardiac arrest team and helping the team as required. You watch all the nurses and doctors immediately taking action to save the person's life and it seems as if they know exactly what to do. Nobody is talking out loud; they are all just 'doing' things. You wonder how they can do this and how they know what the right thing to do is. What you can't see is the nurses or doctors 'reflecting-in-action'. They may be:

- drawing on a number of similar previous experiences
- examining which one is most similar to the one they are now managing
- possibly considering evidence on new medication
- deciding how to manage the environment they are in
- remembering how they felt the last time they had to undertake a similar situation and telling themselves *'this time I am going to manage this well . . . now what do I need . . . I need to keep talking to him as well, even though he is probably not really hearing me . . . hang on, I think I can feel a pulse . . . must mean his heart is now working . . . best tell Dr Bloggs that it is thready and fast though, and I think missing beats as well . . . best get the monitor attached . . . now he is coming round . . . in order to see what his heart trace is doing . . .'.*

In other words, they are using previous knowledge and experiences to influence their actions in the present situation. All of this probably takes place in a very short space of time – but you can see how much reflection-in-action is taking place. Speaking your thoughts out loud is not appropriate in a cardiac arrest situation or in other situations such as breaking bad news. Reflecting-in-action involves private and personal thoughts and feelings.

Banning (2008) suggests that a 'think out loud' approach may be an excellent way to get student nurses to learn as they problem-solve a case study, just as they would in real life practice.

However, reflection-*on*-action requires a set of skills that can be learned, such as self-awareness which is fundamental to learning from experiences in practice, as is being able to recognise what you did well or need to work on should you experience a similar situation in the future. Using a framwork to guide you in writing your reflection of an event or an observation is helpful.

Models/frameworks to help you reflect on practice learning

There are a number of models that can be used based on theories of reflection. We can consider two here that may be useful to you or that your University asks you to use to reflect on your learning.

🔖 Activity

Look at your programme handbook, your personal and professional development document or information in the virtual learning environment at your university. Identify which model or framework is being advocated at the stage of learning you are at. There may also be helpful sheets that you can print out on which to document your reflections of situations or events.

Situations that have a significant impact on your experience and learning are often known as 'critical incidents' – which can be so-called positive or negative situations – hence the word 'critical', in the sense of being important. This is not to be confused with 'critical incident recording' in the clinical area whereby an incident is critical in the sense of being important which has also triggered a serious situation requiring investigation. For example, say a patient had been left on their own in the bathroom when the nurse went to get something. The

nurse didn't make sure there was someone to stay with the patient and they later became dizzy, collapsed and broke their leg. This led to them having to go back to the operating theatre, move to an orthopaedic ward and stay in hospital for a further 2 weeks. Such an incident would have to be reported, written down in a factual way and then signed by the nurse, and subsequently investigated by a senior member of staff.

🔖 Activity

Consider this example of a critical incident and reflect on what happened. What can you infer from the 'second hand' description above, and what do you think would have been the description of the event by the actual nurse in question?

A helpful model for reflecting on practice learning (upon which many others are based) is Gibb's (1988) 'reflective cycle' (see Fig. 14.1).

A simpler version of this model for reflection is that by John Driscoll (1994). His framework is based on three stages: What? So what? And now what?

(See http://www.supervisionandcoaching. com/pdf/reflectivelearning.pdf.)

In brief, you have an experience in practice and then ask yourself the three questions relating to this experience:

1. **What?** This is your account or description of the experience or event that took place, making considered judgements on what you think happened and why it happened (description).

2. **So what?** This is when you consider how you felt and decide if it was a good experience or a bad experience and why. You decide what you think you learnt from the experience or the event (feelings, evaluation and analysis).

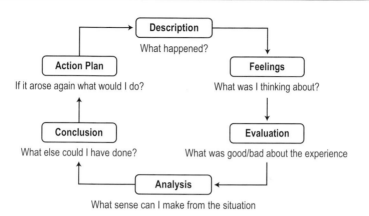

Fig 14.1 The reflective cycle (adapted from Gibbs (1988) with permission)

3. **Now what?** This is where you decide what you are going to do in relation to learning from this experience or event. You decide what actions may be necessary, such as: discussing it with someone else; reporting aspects of the experience officially to another person; or developing your knowledge and skills to manage the situation better or differently next time something similar happens (conclusion and action plan).

Activity

Consider an experience in your surgical placement and use Gibb's and Driscoll's models of reflection. Write the reflective cycle experiences in your reflective diary, which will either be part of your portfolio or part of your personal and professional development document. Discuss this with your mentor and personal tutor (normally a requirement of your programme). If you have to write a critical reflection essay or similar, you may want to read Chapter 4 in Gimenez (2011) (see References).

Establishing knowledge and skills gained in practice

You now have a framework for reflection on practice learning in your surgical placement. From a clinical perspective, it is also important to consider what you have learnt from this book (or individual chapters) and actually caring for patients undergoing surgical interventions.

You may have agreed a learning plan with your personal tutor prior to the placement and discussed it with your mentor, who would then facilitate achievement of the learning plan as far as possible. At the end of your placement, you may have to provide evidence for achieving this or your mentor may have to do so, or both, identifying areas for further development in general and on future clinical placements. An example can be seen in Box 14.1.

Transferrable practice and knowledge

Throughout this book, there are many activities to test your knowledge as you

Box 14.1 Example of a learning agreement for a surgical placement experience

Learning outcome

To assess, plan and contribute to implementing and evaluating the care of a patient undergoing surgery.

Experiences to be gained

1. Exposure to new situations which involve preparation of patients undergoing surgery.
2. Discuss with mentor pre- and postoperative care protocols in place.
3. Assess the needs of a patient who is admitted for surgery.
4. Plan the care and record in the patient care plan under supervision.
5. Obtain and read current research findings on wound care specific to different patient groups.

Criteria for success

1. Should be able to assess the needs and plan the care for a patient undergoing surgery.
2. By demonstrating, under supervision, the total preparation of one patient undergoing surgery.
3. Can give a rationale for three nursing interventions which are linked to current research findings.

All of the above would be agreed with your personal tutor prior to commencing your placement experience and discussed and agreed with your mentor when you meet to discuss your learning needs and goals and how they can support you in achieving them.

Evidence of achievement

1. (Name: e.g. Jane) has assessed and planned the care of four patients during this placement and has 'followed through' two of these from preoperative preparation to the patient being discharged home from hospital. This included a visit to the operating theatre and a day with the stoma nurse.
2. The diary summary for this placement indicates that (e.g. Jane) was distressed by one incident which she also highlighted as a critical incident record (discussed with her).
3. She accepts support and constructive criticism in care planning, then acts upon it in a positive way.
4. She has been able to identify the evidence-base research for three interventions as agreed plus many others (handwashing, preoperative fasting and assessment of pain).

Box 14.1 Example of a learning agreement for a surgical placement experience—cont'd

Areas for further development

1. Needs to discuss with her personal tutor the issues raised within this experience, especially those in the reflective diary records.

2. Her aseptic technique skills need to be extended/applied to many new areas of practice.

3. Very positive attitude to learning and achieving her goals. Main area to develop is writing her reflections on events that can lead to consideration of the role of others in patient care.

---

progress through the patient journey in the perioperative period. The intention of this chapter is to use reflection to help you consider what you have learnt and to offer additional learning exercises to test your knowledge, together with some case scenarios that you can use to develop your notes on all aspects of perioperative care. Some of these may be potential examination questions which can be used for revision purposes.

Self assessment questions: perioperative care

14.1. List 10 possible preoperative care procedures that are necessary to ensure the safe environment of the patient is maintained prior to surgery.

14.2. In the transfer of patients to theatre, what can the nurse do to maintain the safety of the patient?

14.3. Immediately postoperatively, what is the nurse's role in maintaining the safety of the patient?

14.4. List 10 actual or potential problems than could occur postoperatively after major surgery.

(See pages 185–186 for answers.)

The acutely ill adult: planning care following surgery

Case history

Mr William Smith, age 58, was taken to the operating theatre for removal of a large malignant tumour from his large colon. The possibility of a permanent colostomy had been discussed with him and his wife. During the operation, Mr Smith experienced a cardiac arrest which the anaesthetist believed was due to a myocardial infarction (evidence seen on the cardiac monitor). He was successfully resuscitated and the surgeon completed the planned surgery which took longer than planned. He was taken to the recovery room for close observation until the anaesthetist decided when it was safe to transfer him to the ward or, preferably, given the cardiac arrest, a high dependency unit (HDU). Unfortunately, no HDU bed was available at the time so, with reassurance from the ward that they could maintain close 24-hour observation on his progress, the anaesthetist agreed that he could be returned to the ward once his observations were stable and he was awake and responsive.

On his return to the ward, you and your mentor, a staff nurse with intensive care unit experience, were assigned by the team leader to look after him. You had already prepared the bed area for his return and it had been possible to re-allocate him to a small single-bedded room near the nurse's station. His wife and daughter were already waiting for his return and had been informed by the surgical registrar, who had assisted during the surgery, about his cardiac arrest and the need for close monitoring. Despite being distressed by this news, they remained positive about the care he would receive on his return and were pleased that he was coming back to be cared for by staff who knew him.

Specific information you need for the following activity related to the case history

The postoperative plan from theatre for Mr Smith includes the following information (in brief):

- Removal of tumour (malignant as per preoperative investigations); end-to-end anastomosis of large intestine–sigmoid colon (no colostomy formed).
- Cardiac arrest due to myocardial infarction – effects enhanced by the surgical intervention. Successfully resuscitated (2 minutes) and vital signs stabilised. Two-hour period in recovery room.

Instructions for nursing staff regarding observations are as follows:

- Cardiac monitoring to continue, as well as all other observations.
- Pulse and blood pressure: quarter-hourly for 2 hours then reassess; if stable for that 2 hours, nursing staff to determine observations either half-hourly or hourly as other physiological status requires. Continuous re-evaluation as necessary and surgical registrar to be contacted if any changes in cardiac monitoring and function. Cardiac medical team will be

attending the patient to assess myocardial infarction status and long-term rehabilitation needs.

- Patient was slightly hypothermic postoperatively at a temperature of 35.6°C; to restabilise slowly until his 'normal' body temperature is re-established.
- Counteract fluid loss during surgery: he is to have an IV infusion of dextrose/saline and normal saline to alternate every 4–6 hours as blood pressure and fluid output determine.
- For the first 6 hours postoperatively, he requires central venous pressure measurements taken and he will then be reviewed by the anaesthetist who wishes to be kept informed of his general ongoing postoperative status.
- He has a nasogastric tube in situ and aspirations initially are hourly.
- Due to the complications in the operating theatre, he has a catheter in situ as well for 24 hours, until his cardiac problems have been stabilised. Hourly measurements to be taken and recorded.
- He has a patient-controlled analgesia (PCA) machine which he had explained to him preoperatively and the nurses are to monitor his use of it given that he has had the myocardial infarction.
- He has a wound drain in situ and his wound has been closed with clips.

He has been fully conscious on his return to the ward and has been made comfortable, although he is aware that there is a lot of equipment around his bed and he is reluctant to move. He is aware of his condition and his wife and daughter are with him.

◆ Activity

Based on this very brief insight into Mr Smith's physiological status and postoperative situation, consider the following questions and exercises. Use other chapters and resources identified in this book to help you consider all of the issues raised in this scenario and information offered.

- Plan his care in order of priority and use an appropriate nursing model as a framework for his care. Do this for the first 12 hours postoperatively, then 48 hours, then 7 days.
- Determine what equipment you will need in order to ensure his internal and external safe environment.
- Explain the effects of hypovolaemia on the body and how it determines the importance of nursing observations, including how the signs of hypovolaemia would be noted.
- Explain the effects that a myocardial infarction has on the muscle and blood supply of the heart.
- Determine what needs Mr Smith will have problems in meeting during the first 24 hours, 36 hours and 7 days postoperatively.
- How would you and your mentor organise the care of Mr Smith in order to allow:
  - for his safety
  - for your learning experience and gaining competences for meeting the NMC domains
  - for the involvement of all the healthcare team involved in his care?

Discuss this with your mentor as a hypothetical patient situation, but one where you can identify some specific learning needs and goals to achieve in order to establish prior knowledge and skills should a situation like this arise either in your current or future placements.

Transferring knowledge and skills

Whether this is your first placement or your final one, you will be able to use what you have learnt in this surgical placement to help you in either your next placement or in your role as a qualified nurse.

Activity

Make a list of all you have learnt in this surgical placement, and record it as part of your practice achievements in your practice assessment document. Discuss with your mentor how this can contribute to your ongoing record of achievement (NMC 2010). If it is your final placement, you will be assessed by your nominated sign off mentor.

If you are pursuing a programme leading to registration as a nurse in any of the four fields of practice, please refer to the generic NMC domains and competences for identifying how undertaking a surgical placement can be of value in relation to your own specific field of practice and the patients/clients/children/young people/adults that you meet and care for.

Summary

Wherever you are in your stage of learning, it is important to recognise the interdependence of knowledge and skills gained in other placements, the knowledge and skills you learn in the university setting and their application in the reality of clinical practice. This book can help you only as a guide to the possibilities of caring for different patients and in very different surgical placement contexts. Remember, every placement is very different, every day is very different, every patient is very different and every event is very different. You can, however, develop knowledge and skills to enable you to adapt to this uncertain environment and become a competent decision maker and problem solver as well as a caring, knowledgeable student nurse ready to take on the responsibilities of becoming and being a registered nurse.

References

Banning, M., 2008. The think aloud approach as an educational tool to develop and assess clinical reasoning in undergraduate students. Nurse Educ. Today 28 (1), 8–14.

Driscoll, J., 1994. Reflective practice for practise – a framework of structured reflection for clinical areas. Senior Nurse 14 (1), 47–50.

Gibbs, G., 1988. Learning by doing: a guide to teaching and learning methods. Further Education Unit, Oxford Polytechnic, Oxford.

Gimenez, J., 2011. Writing for nursing and midwifery students, 2nd ed. Palgrave Macmillan, Basingstoke.

Hart, S., 2010. Nursing: study and placement learning skills. Oxford University Press, Oxford.

Miller, E., Webb, L., 2010. Active listening and attending: communication skills and the healthcare environment. In: Webb, L. (Ed.), Nursing: communication skills in practice. Oxford University Press, Oxford.

Nursing and Midwifery Council, 2010. Standards for pre-registration nursing education. NMC, London. Online. Available at: http://standards.nmc-uk. org/PreRegNursing/statutory/ background/Pages/introduction.aspx (accessed September 2011).

Price, B., Harrington, A., 2010. Critical thinking and writing for nursing students. Learning Matters, Exeter.

Schon, D.A., 1983. The reflective practitioner. Basic Books, New York.

Timmins, F., 2008. Making sense of portfolios – a guide for student nurses. Open University Press, Maidenhead.

Webb, L., 2010. Nursing: communication skills in practice. Oxford University Press, Oxford.

Further reading

Aston, L., Wakefield, J., McGowan, R., 2010. The student nurse guide to decision making in practice. Open University Press, Maidenhead.

Wilding, M., 2008. Reflective practice: a learning tool for student nurses. British Journal of Nursing 17 (11), 720–724.

Websites

See John Driscoll's Website for resources, including a presentation on reflection to students at the University of Salford and a range of articles: http://www. supervisionandcoaching.com/ (accessed September 2011)

Reflection on Practice: an excellent resource as part of the Making Practice Based-Learning Work project led by the University of Ulster: http://www.science.ulster.ac.uk/nursing/ mentorship/docs/learning/ reflectiononpractice.pdf (accessed December 2011)

Learning and Assessing through Reflection – as above: http://www.science.ulster.ac.uk/ nursing/mentorship/docs/learning/ RoyalBromptonV3.pdf (accessed December 2011)

Online resources from Webb (2010). This is one of a series of books which can help with specific aspects of learning as a student nurse. Most of these have online resources which can be accessed independently but may require some linking to key information in the text itself: http://www.oup.com/uk/ orc/bin/9780199582723/01student/ practice/ (accessed December 2011)

NMC advice on use of social networking sites: http://www.nmc-uk.org/Nurses-and-midwives/Advice-by-topic/A/Advice/Social-networking-sites/ (accessed December 2011)

Answers to self-assessment questions

(Note: these are not *definitive* answers. Please read the relevant chapters for full details.)

14.1

1. Assessment and recording on admission of blood pressure, pulse, respiration and temperature (and note these baseline observations).
2. Urine analysis is undertaken and weight is measured and recorded.
3. Check that the informed consent form has been signed by the patient and is in the patient notes.
4. Procedure site is marked.
5. Check if the patient has been given information and time to ask questions regarding the impending surgery.
6. Check preoperative instructions from the surgeon and all premedication and postoperative medication written.
7. Immediately prior to taking the patient to theatre, check the name band, and that the name and date of birth of the patient in the notes matches the name band and patient response.
8. Any X-rays are with the patient notes.
9. When the patient last ate or drank.
10. Check that any drug or other allergies have been noted either at the pre-admission clinic or on admission to the ward. Allergies recorded in the theatre 'checklist' including latex allergy or specific drugs/antibiotics. Any false teeth removed and any loose teeth recorded, jewellery removed or secured (e.g. wedding ring) so as not to interfere with surgery or to adhere to religious customs, ensure any prostheses are

removed and any nursing and medical records are up to date and complete to go with the patient to theatre. (See Chapter 6 for more details.)

14.2

1. Talk to the patient and reassure.
2. If on a theatre trolley, ensure the patient is unable to roll off the trolley (ensure any trolley side arms are secure to prevent this); if on their own bed, ensure the same thing; ensure arms and/or legs are not hanging over the sides where they may be damaged.
3. Check for any signs of obvious physical distress especially if the patient is sedated or has known cardiac or respiratory problems.
4. On arrival in the anaesthetic room, ensure that the verbal handover includes all information and that you stay with the patient if that would allay further anxiety.
5. All nursing and medical notes and X-rays handed over and checked.

14.3

1. Maintain a safe internal environment:
   - Maintain a clear airway.
   - Correct positioning of patient depending on the surgery.
   - Observations as per anaesthetist request are carried out (in the recovery room and on return to theward):
     - temperature, pulse and respiration
     - blood pressure
     - wound area, drains and drainage
     - intravenous infusion or blood transfusion
     - oxygen requirements
     - pain management.
2. Maintain a safe external environment:
   - Ensure oxygen and suction equipment are available (especially on return to the ward after discharge from the recovery room).
   - Ensure there is an airway set during transfer from theatre and at the bed side.

14.4 (Note: this is in brief and not in any specific order)

- Shock due to pain (neurogenic) or haemorrhage/fluid loss (hypovolaemic) or heart problems (cardiogenic).
- Obstructed airway.
- Inadequate breathing and potential hypoxia.
- Postoperative hypothermia.
- Postoperative pain.
- Vomiting/nausea.
- Dehydration or fluid overload.
- Impaired nutritional status/malnutrition.
- Postoperative anxiety.
- Urine retention.
- Wound haemorrhage.
- Wound dehiscence ('burst abdomen').
- Paralytic ileus.
- Wound infection.
- Deep vein thrombosis.
- Altered body image.
- Skin breakdown in pressure areas of the body.

⚓ Activity

The following books/chapters can be used to check all of these and find out the actions to either prevent or manage these postoperatively. Make notes against each one for your placement file/notebook. This is not a definitive list and needs to be considered against individual patients and the type of surgery they experience. There will be many actual and potential problems related to specific types of surgery discussed in this book.

Amos A, Waugh A (2007) Caring for the person having surgery. In: Brooker C, Waugh A Foundations of nursing practice. Mosby, Edinburgh

Pudner R (2010) Nursing the surgical patient Baillière Tindall, Edinburgh

Wicker P, O'Neill J (2010) Caring for the perioperative patient, 2nd edn. Wiley-Blackwell, Oxford

Appendix Nursing and Midwifery Council (NMC) guidance on professional conduct for nursing and midwifery students (2009)

The four core principles of the code

Your conduct as a nursing or midwifery student is based on the four core principles set out in the code:

1. Make the care of people your first concern, treating them as individuals and respecting their dignity.
2. Work with others to protect and promote the health and wellbeing of those in your care, their families and carers, and the wider community.
3. Provide a high standard of practice and care at all times.
4. Be open and honest, act with integrity and uphold the reputation of your profession.

Make the care of people your first concern, treating them as individuals and respecting their dignity

Treat people as individuals
You should:

1. Treat people as individuals and respect their dignity.
2. Be polite, kind, caring and compassionate.

3. Not discriminate in any way against those for whom you provide care.
4. Recognise diversity and respect the cultural differences,values and beliefs of others, including the people you care for and other members of staff.

Respect a person's confidentiality
You should:

5. Respect a person's right to confidentiality.
6. Not disclose information to anyone who is not entitled to it.
7. Seek advice from your mentor or tutor before disclosing information if you believe someone may be at risk of harm.
8. Follow the guidelines or policy on confidentiality as set out by your university and clinical placement provider.
9. Be aware of and follow the NMC guidelines on confidentiality (available from the NMC Website: http://www.nmc-uk.org).
10. Make anonymous any information included in your coursework or assessments that may directly or indirectly identify people, staff, relatives, carers or clinical placement providers.

11. Follow your university and clinical placement provider guidelines and policy on ethics when involved or participating in research.

Collaborate with those in your care
You should:

12. Listen to people and respond to their concerns and preferences.
13. Support people in caring for themselves to improve and maintain their health.
14. Give people information and advice, in a way they can understand, so they can make choices and decisions about their care.
15. Work in partnership with people, their families and carers.

Ensure you gain consent
You should:

16. Make sure people know that you are a student.
17. Ensure that you gain their consent before you begin to provide care.
18. Respect the right for people to request care to be provided by a registered professional.

Maintain clear professional boundaries
You should:

19. Maintain clear professional boundaries in the relationships you have with others, especially with vulnerable adults and children.
20. Refuse any gifs, favours or hospitality that might be interpreted as an attempt to gain preferential treatment.
21. Not ask for or accept loans from anyone for whom you provide care or anyone close to them.
22. Maintain clear sexual boundaries at all times with the people for whom you provide care, their families and carers.
23. Be aware of and follow the NMC guidelines on maintaining clear sexual boundaries (available from the advice section on the NMC Website: http://www.nmc-uk.org).

Work with others to protect and promote the health and wellbeing of those in your care, their families and carers, and the wider community

Work as part of a team
You should:

24. Be aware of the roles and responsibilities of other people involved in providing health and social care.
25. Work co-operatively within teams and respect the skills, expertise and contributions from all people involved with your education.
26. Treat all colleagues, team members and those with whom you work and learn fairly and without discrimination.
27. Inform your mentor or tutor immediately if you believe that you, a colleague or anyone else may be putting someone at risk of harm.

Provide a high standard of practice and care at all times

Recognise and work within your limits of competence
You should:

28. Recognise and stay within the limits of your competence.
29. Work only under the appropriate supervision and support of a qualified professional and ask for help from your mentor or tutor when you need it.
30. Work with your mentor and tutor to monitor the quality of your work and maintain the safety of people for whom you provide care.
31. Seek help from an appropriately qualified healthcare professional, as soon as possible, if your performance or judgement is affected by your health.

Ensure your skills and knowledge are up to date
You should:

32. Take responsibility for your own learning.

33. Follow the policy on attendance as set out by your university and clinical placement provider.
34. Follow the policy on submission of coursework and completion of clinical assessments as set out by your university and clinical placement provider.
35. Reflect on and respond constructively to feedback you are given.
36. Endeavour to provide care based on the best available evidence or best practice.

Keep clear and accurate records
You should:

37. Ensure that you are familiar with and follow the record keeping guidance for nurses and midwives (available from the NMC Website: http://www.nmc-uk.org).
38. Ensure that you follow local policy on the recording, handling and storage of records.

Be open and honest, act with integrity and uphold the reputation of your profession

Be open and honest
You should:

39. Be honest and trustworthy when completing all records and logs of your practice experience.
40. Not plagiarise or falsify coursework or clinical assessments.
41. Ensure that you complete CVs and application forms truthfully and accurately.
42. Ensure that you are not influenced by any commercial incentives.

Act with integrity
You should:

43. Demonstrate a personal and professional commitment to equality and diversity.
44. Abide by the laws of the country in which you are undertaking your programme and inform your university

immediately if, during your programme, you are arrested or receive any caution or warning or similar sanction from the police.
45. Inform your university if you have been cautioned, charged or found guilty of a criminal offence at any time.
46. Ensure that you are familiar with and abide by the rules, regulations, policies and procedures of your university and clinical placement provider.
47. Abide by UK laws and the rules, regulation, policies and procedures of the university and clinical placement providers with regard to your use of the Internet and social networking sites.
48. Ensure that you are familiar with and follow NMC advice on the use of social networking sites (available from the NMC Website: http://www.nmc-uk.org).

Protect people from harm
You should:

49. Seek help and advice from a mentor or tutor when there is a need to protect people from harm.
50. Seek help immediately from an appropriately qualified professional if someone for whom you are providing care has suffered harm for any reason.
51. Seek help from your mentor or tutor if people indicate that they are unhappy about their care or treatment.

Uphold the reputation of the nursing and midwifery professions
You should:

52. Follow the dress code or uniform policy of your university and clinical placement provider.
53. Be aware that your behaviour and conduct inside and outside of the university and clinical placement, including your personal life, may impact on your fitness to practise and ability to complete your programme.
54. Uphold the reputation of your chosen profession at all times